The Dementia Doula

Preparing for tomorrow while living for today

Wendy Hall

First paperback edition July 2022

Book cover design by Daria DiCieli

Book cover photography by Earthbound Studio

ISBN 978-0-6451185-1-3 (paperback)

www.dementiadoulas.com.au

CONTENTS

PREFACE..1

CHAPTER 1. Where there's a written will there's a way........5

CHAPTER 2. Filling the empty seat at the table...................21

CHAPTER 3. Tailored for the perfect fit.............................41

CHAPTER 4. Gaps that needed filling.................................63

CHAPTER 5. Snapshot of a better day 79

CHAPTER 6. The weight of grief and loss...........................91

CHAPTER 7. Preparing for a better tomorrow...................107

CHAPTER 8. Building a collaborative community.............123

CHAPTER 9. Support as the end draws near.......................147

CHAPTER 10. A new path awaits 163

Notes on Sources...179

Acknowledgments..187

Preface

I am excited to find myself arriving at my next book, one I've wanted to create for many years. I introduce to you *The Dementia Doula*, or as it's been affectionately known for the last few years, Book 2. Book 2 has been so desperate to be written, but I always knew it had its place and it needed to wait its turn. It's been over many years that streams of narrative destined for Book 2 would flow through my mind needing to be captured. As I wrote down the messages and the dialogue, it was always clear where its ultimate destination would be. The first book of the series - *Dementia can't take everything!* would always set the scene for where we needed to head, and *The Dementia Doula* would closely follow with more of a practical approach and application. The first book would always be the why, and the second would continue to explore the why but start to include the how.

The Dementia Doula was always going to have its own important place, a place in the bigger picture. But while it had been itching to exist for the last few years, it needed to be at the right time, a time where those within the industry would be ready to hear the messages it would convey. It needed those wanting to do more in supporting families to acknowledge they were at a crossroad and were ready to be guided in a new direction. What I didn't anticipate was that I wasn't alone on the path and so many had already been seeking a similar road for a long time.

It was important for me not to just create a dialogue that generated enthusiasm but then leave everything else open for interpretation. That's the script so many of us already know too well. It's always been important for me to complete any story I begin. It was important that I did it in such a way that created hope for a better future and connection within the dementia care sector. I've wanted others to see that if we strive to do and be better, we must also leave room for ongoing improvement and growth. This is the only way we stand a chance of meeting the needs of individuals and do so in a way that continues to bring comfort and a sense of hope for anyone impacted by advancing dementia.

The intention of writing *The Dementia Doula* was to build confidence, provide support and guidance and a resource for the way forward. I wanted it to be a trusted friend for those seeking a different path that aligned with the Dementia Doula vision. This is a book that, like *Dementia can't take everything!*, creates a forum for sharing the learnings from the field, but this time it is from the Dementia Doula perspective. I want us, as Dementia Doulas and those who are Dementia Doulas at heart, to share our stories so that we can grow and learn from each other and create an ever-evolving role that will inspire and support so that no one goes through the dementia experience alone.

The idea for this book came from the frustration I felt for people living with dementia and their families but also for care staff who turn up every day, giving their all while receiving little recognition in return. I wrote this with the hope of providing a forum through which Dementia Doulas can feel comfortable in their role, to provide an opportunity to better connect with each other. If we can do that for ourselves then we stand a better chance of connecting with anyone living with dementia and those that surround them. I wanted to bring together a group of unique individuals who carry a passion for dementia care like no other as a true team that others will want to be a part of, a team that others will want in their employ.

As you read this book and gain an insight into the qualities of a Dementia Doula and the passion and uniqueness the role can bring, it is my hope that it becomes like looking in a mirror where you say, 'Wow, she's describing me'. I hope it's reaffirming you as you journey through dementia care OR that it validates the wonderful things you already do for someone living with dementia and their families. Know that by showing up and being you means you truly make a difference, big or small.

The Dementia Doula role is ever evolving, and I would do it an injustice to suggest I could write an A-Z guide in one edition. Instead, this is a guide for getting started with some tips I have learnt along the way. This book is designed to foster that which you may already be aware you have. It will encourage you to step outside of yourself to see the bigger role you can play, bringing greater meaning and connection for those you represent and advocate for every time you enter their space. This is an exciting new and emerging area and together we'll influence this space like never before. In writing this book, I invite you to not only share in 'how' you got to this point but also 'why' you got to this point. We'll explore the world of the Dementia Doula and see if there isn't a seat there waiting with your name on it.

Many of the lessons I've learnt over the years have been through hindsight, from looking back, seeking patterns, and putting together the stories I have been a part of and seen first-hand. The stories I am sharing here have been constants for me over the years. They're stories I know colleagues will connect with and see different faces in their minds with the same scripts. They're stories that once shared can never be forgotten and they matter. They matter to those who lived them. They matter to those who shared in them. They matter to those who learn from them. This is learning on a whole new level and one that doesn't come with a glossary. To bring back a world thought long gone is to honour the past in a way that ensures moments do matter.

1 • Where there's a written will there's a way

'Failure to talk about and plan for death in advance is one of the most significant obstacles to improving the quality of dying'

- Swerissen & Duckett, p.11

Throughout my career, I've witnessed the lonely death of someone living with dementia. This is a time when those surrounding the person have so much to give but don't know how, where families lack support and connection that would see them better prepared for what was to come and better placed to play a more prominent and active part during the advancing stages of dementia. For many years I've witnessed a disconnect between families, aged care staff and the person living with dementia. I've listened to their stories and watched them do their best navigating the advancing stages of dementia all the while seeming lost, feeling helpless and lacking any sense of direction. I've watched families navigate each moment as it presented itself and we, the service providers, continued to tell them what they needed to do and how they should go about it.

As service providers, we knew funding was tight and a cookie cutter service was all there was to genuinely offer.

I would hear families share stories of crossing their fingers and hoping they were providing the best possible care and support, yet all the while knowing they weren't even close. I saw caring and well-intentioned family members feeling distanced from the person they were supporting while at the same time being reassured by the care sector they no longer needed to worry, that the person's care needs would now be provided for them. I questioned myself, why was it that families appeared to be worrying more than ever and saying they felt shut out? Was it because we were continuing to treat people living with dementia as though they were patients in a hospital, being cared for in a way that would cure and fix or at the very least keep them safe?

I watched families blindly supporting their loved one in the best way possible, with the limited resources they had, looking to those around them for support only to find a reassuring smile and words that fell short. I watched those with advancing dementia seemingly distant and disconnected, their world appearing to have stopped, frozen in time, with the world around them continuing to spin without them. It appeared in many ways that they'd died years before their time and that was how those around responded to them. It saddened me that their end-of-life and eventual death experience would ultimately be one experienced alone.

With personal care needs met, those living with dementia missed opportunity for end-of-life rituals, vigils, times where loved ones could remind them how loved they still were and the impact they'd had. The true essence of what it is to live and then die had long been taken from them. There were no chances to say goodbye or to say I'm sorry. How could we, as a system, have for so long, got it so wrong?

Maggie's story …

Maggie's brother, Brian, was admitted to hospital for hip surgery following a fall. During the lengthy operation, extensive cancer was discovered. Brian now faced a future of uncertainty as he was also living with advancing dementia. Brian received good medical care from staff but following the surgery, Maggie and the rest of Brian's family felt a disconnect. They didn't believe that staff understood Brian's experience or perspective and they seemed to lack an understanding of dementia. This was a frustration for family. Because Brian didn't fit the 'normal' profile of a patient, staff appeared unsure as to how to proceed. The family didn't know how they could bridge the divide, or what they needed to do to ensure Brian was getting the best care possible or the specific type of care he required.

Maggie not only felt a disconnect from her brother, but also from staff. She wanted to help them to understand her brother and his needs but wasn't sure how. Staff didn't have time to connect with her and much needed conversations were missed. Maggie just needed someone to talk to, someone who understood the situation they faced, someone who would listen without judgement, someone who wouldn't necessarily fix the situation but someone who could help her, and the rest of the family, put the pieces together in their minds.

What was Maggie meant to do and what was it exactly that she was waiting for? The answers were difficult to find, and the way forward appeared elusive. Hospital staff would ask family what they wanted, knowing Brian was cognitively unaware and unable to grasp the terminal nature of cancer he now faced. This felt like a loaded question which left the family not knowing how to respond. What were the questions being asked of them? Were there real and tangible options they should seriously be considering or were the questions a token sentiment to test where the family were at?

Hospital staff eventually had a conversation with family and said there wasn't much more they could do for Brian. He was now considered to be palliative. What did these words mean to his family? The questions without answers were beginning again. Were they to take him home? If so, could the family manage Brian's care on their own? Would Brian remain in hospital? If so, would staff just move him to another ward or would he stay where he was? Did someone need to be notified of this change in circumstance? Who would take him into residential care, taking into account his complex medical issues?

Brian's family decided to take him home. A hospital bed and supplies appeared in the family home with a palliative nurse visiting to talk family through the clinical side of his care. The nurse was caring and thoughtful, with Maggie and the rest of Brian's family connecting with him instantly, but in the blink of an eye he was gone, off to the next patient on his list and they were left to make it up as they went along. The system had provided all it could, they were as set up as they could be; the rest was now up to them. They made rosters, shopping lists for supplies, they stocked up the alcohol cabinet, knowing they were there for the long haul, or so they thought ... Within 2 weeks, Brian died.

Brian died within a month of his admission to hospital for hip surgery. His family had rallied to support him not knowing or realising how advanced or quickly things were deteriorating and how close to death he'd been all along. They faced each day as it presented itself, not fully understanding what they were doing or how they should be doing it.

The missing pages

Without guidance or a plan for moving forward as a united front, families just like Maggie's, along with staff, have continued to go it alone, often with the person with dementia dying a lonely and unmeaningful death. There is a lack of clear or consistent approaches in place for assisting families and staff in their understanding of how to navigate and prepare for the later stages of dementia, or for having conversations preparing them for what that may look like. There needs to be a better way forward, a path that doesn't leave anyone behind, one that creates a clear direction and prepares everyone for the ultimate role they will play. It was time to think about what a new way might look like and find a natural point from which to begin.

There appeared to be someone missing from Maggie's and Brian's equation who could piece all questions and supports together for families and guide them along the path they were on, someone who could bring a sense of clarity and provide them with the voice they needed for navigating what they faced today and was inevitably coming their way tomorrow. The missing someone is the Dementia Doula. The Dementia Doula role emerged as the missing part of the equation, an independent role that sat in its own lane. A Dementia Doula would bring together the required information for families and package it in such a way that was tailored to their individual situation and circumstances.

A path of certainty

Planning for our futures very rarely includes what we want our final days and months to look like. There's a fear of the unknown or the belief that avoiding the subject will alleviate any unnecessary emotional pain. But even when someone is diagnosed with a life limiting disease such as a type of dementia, it's still not a natural topic for discussion. Research such as Crowther et. al., (2013), suggests that specialised end-of-life care in this area continues to be unequal or non-existent when compared with other life-limiting illnesses. The flow on from this currently means there's an inconsistent approach to building supportive networks around the person to ensure their end-of-life plans are in place or enacted.

The Dementia Doula role was originally created to fill this widening gap and to create a new model of care that would fit seamlessly into the end-of-life-space. It meant as someone moved closer to end-of-life, highly emotive families were better supported and prepared for time critical decision making when timely and tailored palliative care practices were required. The role was designed to provide a coordinated approach and assistance for how the person's wishes, if they'd been captured or documented, were going to be enacted.

Families empowered through the provision of information, education and support, in turn would be better prepared for future decision making, creating their own plan for moving forward. The Dementia Doula role was designed to offer not only a proactive approach but also be responsive and adaptive to the changing needs of all involved. Dementia Doulas would have the capacity to facilitate a team approach between family, staff and the wider community, supporting future decision making which could even include taking the person home for their final hours or days.

The aim was to avoid having emotionally driven conversations that required significant decisions being made within the final hours, days or even weeks of a person's life. The strength of the role was to be in providing those living with dementia the opportunity to express their wishes for end-of-life care and management at a time when they still had capacity and ability to articulate it for themselves.

Impact of missed conversations

As paramedics, it wasn't uncommon to be called to a home where someone was in cardiac arrest, and CPR was commenced on the person. On one occasion while doing chest compressions on an older lady, I looked up at two distraught adult daughters calmly asking them what their mother's wishes were. One daughter said, 'She wouldn't want to be hooked up to a machine or anything', while the other daughter said, 'She would want everything done for her'. Those heartbreaking responses indicated there had never been a conversation of their mother's wishes, nothing was captured and documented. These two grown women should not have been put on the spot like that, but fate had unfortunately decided otherwise. Whenever there was uncertainty in such a situation, a full resuscitation must commence with flow on transport to hospital.

Advance Care Directives

Many people are reluctant or frightened to discuss their end-of-life wishes and this is in part due to the clinical way it's often done or structured. There's also a societal reluctance and stigma attached to talking about death and dying or in looking too far ahead. People living with dementia are no different. I know of a family member admitted to hospital with a serious condition (but not realising it at the time) and being asked then and there, during their time of distress, what their end-of-life wishes were. A necessary conversation but perhaps the timing or delivery was insensitive. When someone advances with their dementia and loses mental capacity it is ultimately up to their next of kin to provide guidance as to the person's wishes about how things should proceed.

Beth's story …

I think back to an older couple I once had as neighbours. The husband had advancing cancer and I'd spoken with his wife, Beth, about calling me if she ever needed anything. When she mentioned in conversation that her husband no longer wanted to be resuscitated when he died, I asked if this had been spoken about with their doctor and formalised in any way. She said it hadn't but was something she would now follow up. 5am one morning and my phone rings with Beth at the end of the line. I said I'd be right over. I saw Beth's husband struggling to breathe and in a state of distress. I quietly asked her whether there'd been a conversation with their doctor. She said there had been and hurried off to find the paper.

I couldn't believe what I saw when Beth handed me a piece of A4 paper with nothing other than words scrawled diagonally through the centre, her husband's name, NFR (referring to - not for resuscitation) and a scrawly signature underneath. That was it. That was the doctor's Advance Care Directive. I looked painfully at Beth and towards her husband and told them we needed to call an ambulance. That scrawly piece of paper would unfortunately not suffice. Her husband knew he needed assistance and unhappily went to hospital. Things were properly sorted following his return with the distressing situation fortunately not repeated.

Planning for what's to come

It's beneficial for all involved when a palliative approach can be implemented at any stage of the disease duration. This process includes the necessary planning and assessment for how care will unfold and be delivered and is the responsibility of a whole team of specialists. It's a team likely to include a General

Practitioner (GP), Dementia Doula, aged care workers, geriatrician or neurologist and any other health care providers. As a team, it should also include families and support persons. It should also consider support from a specialised palliative care service when the person living with dementia's symptoms deteriorate and become more complex.

Part of the planning stage with the team should include discussion about the care to be provided. This should reflect the person with dementia and their family's wishes. Discussion for future options of care might include suitability of home environments, hospital, or a care home setting. Planning should be ongoing and adapt to the time and presentation of the person's dementia. With an understanding of the processes, families should continue feeling comfortable that contingencies are in place to ensure the management and support for the following:

-   Treatment for pain, nausea, vomiting, infection and shortness of breath
-   Any equipment required to assist with care
-   Support links and networks for families
-   Support for emotional, social, cultural and spiritual concerns
-   Counselling and grief support

By keeping families connected through earlier planning for ongoing care, end-of-life considerations become a natural progression for conversation rather than appearing out of the blue. Families are better positioned and feel more comfortable in reflecting on what their wishes for end-of-life might look like for their loved one. It then naturally flows that the Dementia Doula will be by the side of family for the duration of the disease, during the dying phase and then follow up during the time of bereavement. They play a vital role in assisting families in knowing and feeling they did everything possible to enhance quality of life for their loved one. Validation of sacrifices made and losses experienced over many years, and the integral and meaningful role played for the person with dementia, particularly during the final stages, is essential.

Providing support to someone living with advancing dementia isn't always an easy thing to do. Connecting with the person as they attempt to navigate a disease that not only puts huge challenges in the way, but also one that takes away the person's ability to share their needs, their wants and ultimately their wishes can be difficult. The challenges that someone with dementia faces is distressing for those who try to connect. When attempting to bring back a sense of normality, it can often go so wrong. For far too long we've focussed on managing and 'fixing' someone who's doing the best they can to navigate the day-to-day challenges they encounter rather than supporting what they want as an individual.

Acknowledging all that seemed lost

Dementia will always dictate a person's reality but the care we offer and provide will always be up for negotiation. Some years ago, I was watching an Australian current affairs program which was an exposé of aged care in Australia. I teared up with the voices of the carer 'whistle blowers'. I cried when I heard stories of families who said they felt helpless and alone. I cried feeling deeply saddened on hearing the voices and distress of residents who were struggling. By the end I felt numb. Sadly, these stories were not new to me, and I wasn't surprised by anything I heard or saw. I shed tears for the guilt I felt in being a disempowered part of a system that had given up.

I confess, I did have a few self-indulgent hours following the show. I felt down. I felt sad and hated that there wasn't anything someone like me could do. This was a bigger issue that I couldn't tackle alone. What would I do anyway? This was a systemic problem, and it was accepted, blamed on staff shortages and funding. It felt like a losing battle and beyond the capacity of people like me to fix. It highlighted why so many amazing staff move on or leave the sector altogether. They're drained of anything more to give.

Talk is cheap, and action was required urgently. Alone, I couldn't fix the system, but I realised then I could do my part and I knew there were others like me calling for and desperate for real change. We needed to do better. We had to do better. The images I witnessed needed to serve as a reminder of what we were up against but not deter us from the cause. The need was calling for the development of something that would later become the Dementia Doula role, to fill the space where nothing else existed. The faces they showed were the faces of those we serve, and it was for them we needed to continue showing up for every day, remembering that the person with dementia and their families don't get the option of giving up. They still wake each morning with the same disease and same set of circumstances. They don't get the option of saying 'it's all too hard, I don't want to play anymore'. They live it. It was clear there was a need for a new way forward, and the opportunities suddenly appeared endless.

It was then about finding that starting point, exploring what change could look like and discovering what it might mean to an individual impacted by advancing dementia. It was continuing to search for hope within the ongoing flow of negative stories being generated. It was important not to promise anything that had been promised many times before but not delivered on. It needed to be a direction that would address not just the complexities of navigating future care but also begin to heal hearts broken almost beyond repair. We needed to stop saying 'we'll do better' without providing a definition of what that would look like and avoid setting an unrealistic benchmark that could never be lived up to, one that would fall short and always disappoint.

We needed to go back to the beginning, to start again, to avoid more Band-Aid solutions, and avoid shallow promises that couldn't be believed. We needed to begin rebuilding trust not as a system but as individuals. Things had to change, and this continued to be an itch I needed to scratch, a need to create something, a need to build something, a need to be someone different. How could I fill the gap I continued to see widening? The answer I'd been searching for presented itself in the most unassuming way and was delivered in a fashion I felt was bundled up neatly just for me. The direction I knew I needed to take followed a defining moment when attending an International Dementia Conference.

Pearl's story ...

I sat in the large auditorium as a wife on stage spoke of a specific moment in time she'd experienced with her late husband. I was instantly captivated by the simplicity of her story. It wasn't a novel in the making, and it would unlikely result in a research paper. What Pearl spoke of was her 'most lonely experience'.

Pearl spoke of an experience with her late husband during a hospital admission for advancing cancer, while also experiencing the later stages of dementia. She recounted, with sadness, the loneliness and helplessness she felt being left on her own, sitting by the bedside of her dying husband. Pearl and her husband were left alone for his final days and hours, as it was perceived by staff there was nothing more they could do for him. As she relived the isolation she felt, Pearl was asked by the host what her final take home message for the audience would be. Pearl took a deep breath and simply replied, 'Just be kind'.

Unexpected Pearl of wisdom

For me it was like a lightning bolt from nowhere. Those words, so simple in nature, resonated within me in a way I couldn't have imagined. Those words represented a common need in all of us, for others to show us kindness and empathy, especially in our time of greatest need. At no stage had Pearl asked for a cure or an easy road forward. What she craved for herself, and her husband, was kindness. All she had wanted was for someone to be by their side. My heart broke for them both, knowing such a simple request had not been honoured in her husband's final days. The perception by staff was that nothing more could be done or offered. Oh, how wrong they were!

Where to head next?

My head was spinning. This story was being repeated day after day, year after year. Why? There was no mention in Pearl's story implying staff had been incompetent. It can only be assumed these were highly trained individuals in a busy hospital setting, prioritising their time and resources to those that could be treated or saved. They were unlikely to have specialised dementia training or the environment within which to support someone dying with dementia. Their shift unlikely had time for connection, understanding or compassion. This came at the time where anyone living with a life limiting disease such as cancer would automatically have received specialised and tailored palliative care services while alongside them those living with dementia would continue to go without.

Pearl helped me realise I needed to go back to the basics. My next step was beginning to emerge, and I knew there needed to be a new role moving forward and one I'd need to create. I wasn't sure exactly what it would look like; I lacked clarity at that point in time, but what I did know was that the role would not only offer support for those impacted by advancing dementia but also play a significant advocacy role that could bring to the forefront that which was important to family and be a voice for those without one. This was the person Pearl inadvertently described had been missing for them.

This would be a role created after many years hearing and seeing the pain and disconnection of those impacted by advancing dementia, the battles they stepped up to and faced alone, every single day. It would be a new type of care role that would bring support and tailored palliative care services to anyone with dementia who needed it. While there was no exact science to developing this concept, it would be firmly based on the needs of someone with dementia and their family to be heard, for someone to take time to listen, to hear their stories from their perspective, to hear the hidden pain from those continuing to turn up and do their best every day.

Question for reflection …

What might it feel like being disconnected from the world and those you love when facing an isolating medical condition?

The gift …

When we take time to listen and truly hear, the opportunities become endless.

It broke my heart near the end when I would turn up to visit my husband and find his bedroom door shut and his cries muffled through the shut door. The noise had obviously got too much for staff to bear. To think how frightened and alone he was during that time and there was nothing I could do about it.

• Wife of husband with dementia •

2 • Filling the empty seat at the table

'... many people with advanced dementia are not routinely being assessed to determine their palliative care needs ...'

- Fox et al., 2018 p.1

Dementia care has evolved through reliance on a medical framework that largely influences how people living with dementia are considered. As a physical condition resulting in damage to brain cells, impact on the person differs depending on where in the brain the damage occurs. With over 100 different causes of dementia, this highlights the need for any service delivery to be flexible and adaptable throughout the duration. No two people will experience dementia the same, so moving forward with a new concept meant that services would need to be individually tailored to meet the needs of not only the person with dementia but also their support providers.

Bringing the role to life

Connecting with someone newly diagnosed with dementia and their families is not always easy to do. Many close ranks, shut the world out and try to deal with everything themselves. Alone and frightened, or in denial of the possibilities of an uncertain future where their loved one may be taken away, many families navigate this disease on their own and are left wondering how it will play out for them.

It's often at a time of crisis or rapid and significant decline, when everyday life starts getting more difficult, or a primary carer experiences their own debilitating event, that assistance is sought. When this happens, precious planning time is lost, services come into play in a reactive and responsive way, assistance provided in a time-critical manner with reduced options or pathways. The way forward is directed by services available on the day with decisions made during a time of heightened emotion.

This is a time where there is no offer of hope. There is no sugar coating of how the future will, with a diagnosis of dementia, likely unfold. There is no offer that things may turn out ok. At the beginning, the person and their family are not offered a lot. And when they are, it is commonly a time of information overload, the bundling up of brochures and links to complex websites often difficult to navigate, all whilst in a state of shock and confusion. Lists of support services to contact and other information is hard to digest. What's missing during this overwhelming stage is a starting point, someone to slow things down, to encourage a deep breath and the reassurance that they're not alone.

Challenges to be conquered

Creating a new role in dementia care and bringing it to life was always going to come with challenges. I wondered if others within the aged care field would potentially question the practicality of such a role as a Dementia Doula given the End-of-Life Doula role already existed. I knew the importance of convincing others of the need for an independent and stand-alone role not incorporated into an existing model of care. Due to the simplicity of the role I wanted to create, I kept waiting for someone to say that something similar already existed. Part of me wanted to believe that was possible, that there was something out there I'd not heard of yet or seen people tap into. But there was nothing. Those experiencing advancing dementia were continuing to miss out on palliative specific services that were offered to those without dementia.

Families needed to be part of the bigger picture. They needed to feel this to influence the changes they would ultimately want to see enacted. Aged care continued to be an area that remained over clinicalised and brought with it a strong resistance to change. My hope was to ultimately create a professional role, based on non-clinical principles, that would be respected and bring credibility and value to the aged care field, a role that would be seen to provide a complementary service to those already in place.

Taking on a life of its own

Taking the Dementia Doula concept and bringing it to life was for a long time only something I could imagine. There needed to be a way to capture what it was to be a Dementia Doula and mould it into a shape recognisable by others. This was a role with many facets to it, yet it still sat neatly within the compassionate care sphere, a trusted role that others would call on at times to find a listening ear but to also know that someone could hear their pain, and just be by their side, someone who could assist them to bottle up their wishes and ensure their voices were heard. The Dementia Doula needed to be there supporting and nurturing the person with dementia in their later stages while creating a community of care that wrapped around them and their family for the duration.

This was a role that needed to reflect latest thinking and research and one that supported the need for an independent and autonomous role, one that would work with clients and their families throughout the life limiting disease progression. This was a role that would fit seamlessly into an existing gap, a gap which saw someone with dementia going it alone, isolated, and disconnected from informed family input and connection to appropriate care. It would fill a long-standing need within the community, acute and residential sectors for people living with dementia. Without this tangible role, the palliation stage of the disease process would continue to be missed until the very end even though dementia has a relatively predictable trajectory.

The creation of a dementia specific and independent end-of-life role would strongly impact an area traditionally influenced by the medical field due to no other viable options being available. The flow on effect from this often results in unnecessary hospital presentations and admissions which in turn take up much needed hospital beds. The added undue distress caused to someone with dementia due to these ongoing changes in environments and staffing needed to stop. There was a widening gap between knowledge of best practice in palliative cancer and dementia care and the application in everyday clinical practice.

An autonomous role would have the capacity to connect with families from time of diagnosis through to the bereavement stage which could be over the course of up to 10 years and beyond. This needed to be a role created and designed to be there for the long haul. It couldn't be a service that ceased when funding stopped, or a client reached a particular milestone. For too long I had witnessed first-hand the consequences of a valued service losing funding or have specific access criteria that then saw the service being taken away from a person at a time when they needed it most, leaving them starting all over again: starting again with new faces, new environments, and a new set of rules.

While I began to see small wins along the way, I knew there was more to be done. This was a space that needed significant change and influence in a way never before thought possible. A palliative approach for someone living with dementia needed to be more than just keeping them clean, fed, watered and with a roof over their heads. There was a person trapped inside, within the walls of dementia that had a voice that needed to be heard. The Dementia Doula role was coming to life in a way that could finally be visualised by those that needed it most and people were already knocking at the door.

Creating a concept

I continued researching what the role might look like and where it would comfortably fit. I spoke with specialists, health professionals, colleagues, and care staff along the way. I shared in their frustrations that the palliation stage for people living with dementia wasn't being recognised or identified early enough to meet the person's needs. There were no clearly defined processes for putting in place a palliative approach, for supporting the person and their family as death drew nearer. There was no speed dial to palliative care services or a clear understanding of what they could offer.

Collectively their concerns continued to flag a gap where those with dementia were missing access to vital services along with someone to take the lead ensuring everyone was on the same page. Palliative care is a specialised treatment, care and support regime for people living with a life-limiting illness. It will have been determined they're unable to be cured and it's likely to be the illness they will die from. Palliative care also supports family and friends and aims to ensure a good quality of life. While this type of care is automatically put in place for someone with a diagnosis like cancer, there isn't the same consideration when it comes to dementia.

Having worked for many years in pre-hospital, community, hospital, and residential settings, I could see the missing links in so many areas for people with dementia and their families. The person diagnosed often found themselves caught up in what could only be described as a whirlwind. While they would likely have known for some time that changes were happening, and that something wasn't right, the reality was something quite life shattering. Life as they knew it, from that point, would never again be the same and they were fully aware of the consequences, when plans and dreams for the future all came crashing down. I would continue to witness the loneliness of dementia, not because there was no one around, but because they were surrounded by others trying to control the uncontrollable. As I searched for a suitable model to base the concept on, the role of the End-of-Life Doula presented itself to me even more prominently as a family member went through palliative care.

End-of-life Doulas were becoming more popular within the palliative field, but it was widely known that tailored palliative services hadn't historically been offered to someone with advancing dementia and this seemed a logical model to explore. The End-of-Life Doula is a non-clinical role providing support and guidance for someone with a life-limiting disease, along with their family, during the last 12-18 months of life. The role in its current form didn't offer services specifically for someone with end stage dementia. The end-of-life phase of dementia can be difficult to determine, and the timeframe difficult to ascertain.

While the End-of-Life Doula model ticked many of the necessary boxes, I could see there was more that could be included to meet the specific needs generated by dementia. What seemed to be a good fit was the term Dementia Doula. By narrowing the scope of the role to focus primarily on dementia, this new role would provide an individualised and tailored service specialising in dementia. But why the term Doula? The definition of a Doula is, 'A professional who provides support and assistance to individuals or families, especially during a medical or emotional crisis (used in combination): end-of-life doulas who offer comfort and companionship to dying patients' (dictionary.com 2022). So really, it was the obvious path.

The starting point for the Dementia Doula role was to review services offered when someone with dementia was actively palliating and likely residing in residential or supported type of care. As the role started to build, it became evident that this was a service that should be offered much earlier in the dementia trajectory. When someone is newly diagnosed with dementia, they're effectively told they have a life limiting disease right from the start, that there is no hope for a cure at that point in time. This was a service that could be offered while the person continued to reside within their own home, a time when future considerations could include the person themselves.

The Dementia Doula would ultimately be a specialized role supporting current palliation practices and become the voice of the person and their family. It would also connect by guiding staff who would have little to no understanding of dementia as a disease process or how to incorporate a palliative care approach into care provision. This specialty role would bridge the gap between non-clinical and clinical care and ensure consistency of service received by the person with dementia. The Dementia Doula would seamlessly integrate into the residential, acute and community sectors and play a key role in providing support, education and advocacy for clients, family, and staff. Clients would then be presented with more options including the opportunity to either remain or return to their home environment for the final stage of the disease process.

The Dementia Doula role creates an exciting new career pathway that has at its core components of care that attracted many of us to the health and aged care field in the first place - a pathway that utilises the skills, knowledge and practice of staff who play a strong advocacy role for those they currently support. The role can bring increased job satisfaction and entice staff to stay within the industry rather than leave through lack of options. It is a long overdue role that stands by the family and ultimately the person themselves. It is a role that gives passionate staff an opportunity to do and be more for the individual and provide the opportunity to educate, support, influence and create a community of connection and compassion. It is a role that ensures the final months or years are experienced in true comfort, peace and ensures no one dies alone.

Stepping into the shoes of a Dementia Doula

The role of Dementia Doula was created to fill the need for a non-clinical and independent practitioner with specialised compassionate care expertise. The Dementia Doula would be there to guide family and staff in not only identifying the palliation stage earlier but also supporting a shifting away from ineffective 'active' treatments while focussing on the benefits of a holistic comfort care approach. (Active treatments are those recommended for providing a cure or sustaining life while a body heals or recovers. It's intended to restore the person to a previous health status.) The Dementia Doula is needed to assist all parties involved in navigating the appropriate services required and to ensure the implementation of tailored end-of-life care with a focus on comfort and connection.

A Dementia Doula was never intended to just be a service or program. It was always intended to be someone, a real person, prepared to stand up for and be by the side of those who need them most. They would get everyone on the same page creating a clear understanding of what was happening today and preparing all for what was to come. They would assist families in coming together to work out a plan, a plan where everyone had a designated loosely defined role, one that would be ever changing and adaptive to the needs of the day, for issues big or small. The Dementia Doula would support anyone impacted by advancing dementia in moving forward through the ever-changing landscape together as a united front.

There was suddenly an opportunity to influence and create a role based on what had been wished and hoped for over many years; a role built from the ground up, ensuring it encompassed the 'why' and never losing sight of the bigger picture and greater cause. This would be a role built on the need to serve and serve it would. There was finally an opportunity to provide a dignified approach to the final stage of dementia care.

Benefits of the role

As a non-clinical role focusing on the implementation of a holistic palliative approach for someone with dementia, the Dementia Doula:

- Initiates and facilitates earlier conversations about advance care planning
- Promotes earlier implementation of more timely, appropriate and tailored palliative care practices, especially during the last 12-18 months of life

- Provides staff and family guidance in understanding the definition of 'active' treatment and the consequences that will likely follow
- Focuses on the promotion of holistic palliative comfort care.
- Provides support and guidance for someone with dementia and their families
- Bridges the gap between non-clinical and clinical care practices
- Seamlessly integrates into the residential, acute and community sectors
- Provides support, education and advocacy for clients and staff

Difference between the Dementia Doula and End-of Life Doula roles:

While many similarities exist between the two roles, there are key areas that distinguish them and make the Dementia Doula role quite unique. While an End-of-Life Doula can provide a doula service to someone living with dementia, Dementia Doulas have received specialised and comprehensive training for the provision of a specialised service, a service tailored towards the uniqueness and diversity that comes with dementia. The Dementia Doula role could be likened to a trained general nurse who has chosen to undertake further study and specialise within a specific area offering a higher level of service and care. Key differences include:

Dementia Doulas:

- Generally work within aged care, community and home environments
- Longer trajectory within the life-limiting phase, possibly up to 10 years
- Services can be initiated from time of diagnosis and remain in situ for many years

- Work with aged care staff, clinicians, specialists, GPs and families
- Assist in recognising the transition to the terminal phase of the disease
- Works with the person with dementia early to provide choice and input into future care
- Provide support for family to speak on the person's behalf and initiate treatment and care provision
- Provide support so families are more involved in care for longer
- Have a comprehensive understanding of the aged care industry

End-of-Life Doulas:

- Work generally within hospitals, hospices, and home environments
- Have a shorter trajectory working with the life limiting phase, more likely to be within the last 12-18 months of life
- Work with hospital and hospice nursing/medical staff
- Are more involved with palliative care teams and families where the end stage of life is more easily identified
- Ensure the patient has input into care provision and wishes until later in disease or illness
- Encourage family to play a support role for enacting patient's wishes for treatment and care
- Have a shorter involvement during the terminal phase
- Have a comprehensive understanding of hospitals and palliative care

It was evident that the End-of-Life Doula principles (Krawczyk & Rush, 2020) would provide a solid foundation from which the Dementia Doula role could continue to grow, helping with the creation of a more structured framework on which to build and provide more understanding of the role within the dementia context. The Dementia Doula is there in a specific capacity to advocate, to listen, to advise of rights, to build confidence for conversations and make space for ongoing dialogue. There is a clear defining scope for the role, and it doesn't include entering into care home politics, medical or clinical issues, or personal care issues other than to listen and ensure clients feel heard.

Uniqueness of the role

The Dementia Doula is a unique and specialised role. I'll compare the service offered by a Dementia Doula with a personal experience you may connect with - and one I've lived first-hand.

While I don't profess to know what it's like to have dementia, I do know what it's like to try navigating services, to be left flustered and annoyed, trying to access something without knowing exactly what it might look like or what it's actually called, being left feeling incompetent and useless. It's like me wanting to buy a new computer. Now, I don't know anything about computers, so when I need a new one, I just need a new one. The timing is likely to be inconvenient and a deadline likely looming.

I go to the store and speak with a salesperson who asks me what I want and what I want it to do. I just want a computer. They provide information for which I have absolutely no understanding. All I want is a computer. They direct me to brochures to read about capabilities and size which, firstly, I don't have time for and, secondly, I still don't get what they're talking about. All I want to know is which computer will be the best for me. Is there one I can walk out with right now, that's ready to go? I just need a computer. I leave in frustration and likely close to tears. I speak to a friend in passing about my issue and they say they've just bought a new computer. They tell me the brand and model and I query whether they're happy with it. I ask if it does what they need. Is it easy to navigate? When they reply, 'Yes', I go straight out and buy that computer. I don't know if it's the best computer for me, but the process often becomes so overwhelming I end up taking the easiest option.

Now think about navigating services for someone with dementia. Who is there helping them to navigate the early and later stages of the disease and the in between? Who is there assisting them with options available to them? Who helps narrow down the information, the brochures, the website links so it's easily understood, so it's not so overwhelming? Who presents the information needed for the unique situation they now find themselves in? No one fills this space on a daily basis. Staff in existing roles do amazing work but are often over stretched on a day-to-day basis, trying to be everything to everybody, trying to tick all the boxes that they're required to tick.

What's been missing is the Dementia Doula, someone with the sole purpose of streamlining what's going on, to direct and devise a plan for where everyone's headed and how they're going to get there. They're there for the good, the bad and the undecided, the chaotic, the calm and the sadness. The earlier this relationship is established, the more supported families feel and the better understanding they have of the path ahead.

The Dementia Doula becomes the consistent approach needed by anyone impacted by the effects of advancing dementia. They help take away the guilt and doubt and allow families to just be who they're meant to be, wives, husbands, daughters, sons, grandchildren, with a plan in place so family can take on whatever role they want and feel most comfortable with.

Qualities of a Dementia Doula

The Dementia Doula is someone with a strong desire and passion for supporting those impacted by dementia in a way that enables them to be heard. They're flexible and adaptable, and at times, required to make it up as they go along. They see families as being as impacted by dementia as the client is themselves. They strive to keep families connected and informed. They are the conduit through which families receive information in a digestible format at a time when it's of most relevance. They take their lead from the family unit ensuring everyone stays onboard.

Dementia Doulas enter the lives of families when they are often at their most vulnerable and navigate this time with care and compassion. They may enter the lives of families at any time throughout the disease continuum and can pick up and lead from that point in time. They provide a continuity of service and guidance every step of the way. These qualities are often limited within community based, home based, residential and hospital settings.

A Dementia Doula places families in the driver's seat. They help families to navigate the trajectory of dementia, to get from point A to B. Following a dementia diagnosis, families are encouraged to connect with a Dementia Doula for guidance sooner rather than later to ensure they feel supported for the duration. A significant aspect of the role lies in building safe, supportive and protective communities around the person with dementia and to do so in such a way where everyone's briefed and aware of what the person's going through and how they can best provide connection and support.

The services of a Dementia Doula are not likely to be required constantly throughout the dementia journey, but knowing they are there, waiting in the background for when they're needed most, can bring families an ongoing sense of comfort and reassurance. This consistent approach alleviates families being placed in chaotic situations when a catastrophic event ultimately occurs. The Dementia Doula works with families to create their own individualised plan, so they're better prepared for what's to come and who they want by their side supporting them. A Dementia Doula is aware they can't be everything to everybody but still provide an important service that's valued by those they connect with, a service that meets them where they're at and not where it's thought they should be.

A Dementia Doula brings dementia into the public domain in a way that starts a long overdue conversation with the broader community, connecting others to the experience of dementia in a way they'll understand and relate to, regardless of their individual circumstances. They create a dialogue that ultimately normalises dementia in a way those experiencing it so desperately crave. The Dementia Doula creates an opportunity for people with dementia to link into tailored palliative care practices in a way they currently don't have access to. By moving aspects of dementia care away from a medicalised model of care, there is space to create a community around the person at a time when they're at their most vulnerable.

Jim's story ...

A few years ago, I was tasked with a job that fell outside my normal scope as a Dementia Educator. I was sent to work with staff of a care home refusing to allow the admission of a new resident named Jim. Staff were aware of his 'aggressive' tendencies and these stories put them all on edge. Because of the geographical location, Jim had spent the previous 6 months in a hospital bed awaiting placement to an available care home bed. I travelled with a colleague to the hospital where she collected Jim's belongings. My role at the time, was to convince staff it was a good idea that they should take on his ongoing care.

We arrived at the hospital to find a security guard at Jim's door. With sadness I could only imagine the mixed messages this would send to someone with dementia, as well as the stigma and embarrassment felt by family. I wasn't sure how I would tackle this, when the answer presented itself before my very eyes. As my colleague walked from Jim's room, she carried his belongings, including a stack of photos in frames. What caught my eye was a framed portrait photo of Jim in his military uniform, a distinguished young man who had sacrificed all for his country. I wondered if this was the key I needed to unlock the resistance he unknowingly faced from care home staff.

I asked my colleague to borrow the portrait. As I prepared to speak with 30 plus staff, I placed the photo of Jim front and centre and stood next to it for the duration. I spoke to the photo as though Jim had joined us for the conversation. I spoke of Jim in a way that looked beyond his dementia. Of the 30 plus staff before me, only two had met him in person. I was gifted the opportunity to bring Jim to life so that staff could see him for who he was and what he was, what he stood for and what he was prepared to fight for. His current responses to the darkness of a nightshift and towards anyone who suddenly appeared in front him took on a whole new meaning. They could now see a soft-hearted man who would respond in what appeared to be an aggressive manner when frightened. They finally saw a man they believed they could connect with.

Dementia Doulas bring someone to life in a way that connects others and assists them to see past the dementia, to help navigate and make sense of the responses and where they're likely coming from. While not everyone was sold on the idea, there was marked decrease in resistance for Jim's relocation. The caring nature I tapped into within staff meant they knew he needed their help. The manager contacted me later to share that following the session, three staff members not only approached and said to him Jim was now welcome but asked to work directly with him.

Bringing together the care needed was about coordinating all involved and getting them on the same page. In Jim's case, it was about utilising the resources provided by family and obtaining a thorough history of his life. It was working with staff collectively and bringing Jim to life in such a way they could better connect, then work with management to ascertain why particular staff had an issue with Jim and how this could be resolved. A response to the needs of someone living with dementia will never fully be maximised unless there's a coordinated approach in place.

Dementia Doulas positioned front and centre

Dementia Doulas are committed to setting a new benchmark within the aged care sector by placing the person living with dementia at the centre of their practice and all considerations. It's a role that never loses sight of where it fits, prioritising what is important to those impacted by dementia in any given moment. A Dementia Doula combines aspects of care that currently happen ad hoc when time permits, with more formalised palliative care practices. This is a role that I and so many other staff within aged care have been describing as needed for such a long time. It's provided the capacity for us as individual practitioners to finally contribute in a way we knew to be missing. The Dementia Doula role is one that finally brings with it a new job opportunity within the aged care sector, one with choice and ongoing recognition.

Benefits of a Dementia Doula within an existing staffing model:

For people with dementia and families:

- Decrease rate of unnecessary active treatment administration
- Decrease rate of unnecessary hospital presentations
- Bridging clinical and non-clinical components of palliative care to the dementia context
- Supporting staff with end-of-life practices in end stage dementia
- Consistency of palliative care practices and more timely application
- Palliative approach options discussed earlier with families
- Provision of regular and ongoing education sessions for families and staff
- Formation of dementia specific family support groups
- Support and advisory connection for family members

For the aged care industry:
- A new career path opportunity for existing staff
- A career path for attracting staff to the aged care industry
- Increased staff retention
- An autonomous role with capacity to also support staff
- A professional role complementing the roles of other health professionals
- Increased job satisfaction

Question for reflection ...

How do families currently prepare for end-of-life decision making? Whose responsibility is it to initiate?

The gift …

When we move away from a one size fits all approach, connection takes on a whole new meaning.

It's just all so confusing

• Family Member •

3 • Tailored for the perfect fit

'The ability to deliver care that is compassionate, kind and humanistic exists along a continuum across care settings'

- Crowther et al., 2013, p.492

When creating the Dementia Doula role there was a need for a model of care to underpin it, one supported by existing research and established practices. It needed to provide a specialised but flexible framework incorporating a more relationship-centred care approach (Soklaridis et. al., 2016). It would be based on the care that care staff were wanting to provide but lacked opportunity through lack of time and resources. This model needed to have capacity for empowering families in an area where disconnection and guilt were most prevalent. It needed to provide a more formalised and intentional approach and be best placed for informing the direction a Dementia Doula needed to take.

It was important that the model supported the Dementia Doula role in the type of care it provided. It needed to ensure the role had its own unique fit and never competed with the services offered by others but instead complemented their work, enhancing the overall experience for any client. It finally clicked, and I could see not only what was missing but also the space where it would sit. I could see that clinical care and personal care were adequately covered and prioritised, but compassionate care only existed in an ad hoc way.

The Compassionate care model emerged and wasn't only just a good fit but aligned perfectly with other critical areas of care, honouring the wishes of the person and family while supporting aged care staff in the process. Compassionate care was no longer going to be considered something nice to have. It was now going to be an absolute necessity. It reinforced the sense of needing to be more and to do more *for* the person with dementia rather than doing *to* them.

Compassionate care model

The Compassionate care model requires a Dementia Doula to develop an understanding of the values of others and establish a relationship with them. It's responding in a way that's meaningful for a person as an individual and not just as a resident or patient. Compassion can be defined as that which we feel during relationships with others. It's when we involve residents and patients in their own care, asking their preferences, and adjusting actions to meet them where they're at. Compassionate care requires us to personally understand and respond to the pain experienced by another by taking action to do something to reduce it. It shouldn't be mistaken for kindness which can be seen as an act or gesture done with a feeling of goodwill. Compassion runs much deeper and connects with a personal emotion; it's in the ability to understand the emotional state of another person, to put oneself in their shoes. It comes with a much stronger feeling which encourages a Dementia

Doula to do something to alleviate or reduce the suffering being experienced.

Compassionate care may sound like an easy practice to just put in place, set and forget, but it's far more complex than that. It requires a commitment to ensure it doesn't just fall by the wayside or get hidden under or behind everyday practices. Compassionate care has a significant place in health and aged care and especially for those impacted by advancing dementia. It's a known and effective treatment for decreasing changes in behaviours in anyone it connects with. It brings a sense of well-being to all who use it and its adaptiveness to any setting or environment is testament to its effectiveness. It's a tangible treatment that's safe to use in large doses and the best part is, it doesn't come with any nasty side effects.

Compassionate care in its existing form was an area not formalised in any way. It was here that important dialogue should have been taking place, conversations that those within the broader medical field were assuming someone, somewhere along the line had already had with families. There were assumptions families knew what was coming, where they were heading and that everyone within the family unit was onboard. What the person with dementia ultimately wanted didn't exist or was of little consequence. It was assumed families were as ready as they possibly could be given the complexities of dementia. Unfortunately, they didn't know and were far from ready for what lay ahead.

It was often the small special moments that would tend to get lost in all the rush of a nursing shift. With the Dementia Doula, this was now going to change. There was a clear way forward for connecting family, significant others and staff to the person with dementia, and to do so better than we'd ever done before. This was now a way to incorporate new elements to dementia care provision which included playing a strong advocacy role for both the person with dementia and their family. We were creating a role that could be the voice for those without, a voice needed at a time when they desperately needed to be heard.

The Compassionate care model supports a Dementia Doula, providing an opportunity to tap into intuitive and instinctive practices without compromising care provision - to be in tune with what is happening around the person. Often, it's the unspoken things that say so much and provide the cues for where to head and what to say next - to appreciate the moment someone is in and meet them where they are at. These moments can, at face value, appear inconsequential and often missed. But when they are shared with another, they can provide a connection that changes everything.

Just a walk in the park …

I was recently out walking my dog when I stopped at the top of a wooden walkway to allow an older man to finish his climb to the top. He was taking things slowly, and I didn't want my dog to accidently bump him on the way down. When he reached the top, he looked at me and with a breathless smile said, 'That's the first time I've climbed it without holding onto the rails.'

I congratulated him on what was obviously a great achievement and stayed a moment longer to enjoy this triumphant moment with him. It made me smile to hear how proud he was following a double knee replacement. He referred to it as a small milestone, but it was so much more: a moment that would have been missed if I'd missed the cues.

A Dementia Doula now assists those impacted by advancing dementia to navigate an otherwise emotionally complicated process and empowers them to direct their own care in a way that best reflects their wishes. There is a way to share in sensitive and honest conversations. By being in the moment with families, a Dementia Doula can finally plan for tomorrow then bring families back to today, to return them to the present and continue living their best lives. The exciting part has been connecting with others who knew this was their path too.

"Compassion originates as an empathic response to suffering, as a rational process which pursues patients' wellbeing, through specific, ethical actions directed at finding a solution to their suffering ...

– 2016 literature review published by the National Centre for Biotechnology –

When Compassionate care enters the room

Compassionate care is a model that supports a Dementia Doula in their practice, providing an opportunity to listen to the wishes of clients while working alongside their family members, to be sensitive to their beliefs, treat them with dignity and ensure they don't die alone. This was something I'd not seen formalised in my practice, but interestingly, these were the practices I had longed to provide. They were practices I knew my colleagues were addressing in an ad hoc and undervalued way. Compassionate care was not only the missing piece for residents or clients but also for fellow practitioners.

By identifying the existing gaps, necessary change can finally come to life in a tangible way. What is becoming increasingly evident is that families, along with care home staff, continue to feel overwhelmed and disconnected from the end stage of life of the person they are supporting. A resident in the advanced stages of dementia is never going to be offered a bed in a hospice care unit and is unlikely to receive specialised palliative care or tailored treatment and support. While not fitting the hospice criteria for admission, it's also thought someone with dementia residing in a care home setting will already be having their care needs met. Staff in these settings will continue to be left to navigate end-of-life for their residents without any specific training or resources. Care home staff aren't normally equipped to provide such specialised care with the default being good, generalised care delivery, unaware of the needs good end-of-life dementia care requires.

The Compassionate care model provides an opportunity for a Dementia Doula to bring passionate individuals together, coordinated by a single role, creating a supportive community around the person with dementia, so they know they are loved and not alone. It provides the opportunity for conversations to be had at a time when emotions aren't heightened, a time when shared information can be more easily understood and processed, a time when urgent decision making isn't required.

Annette's story ...

The term 'active treatment' is a very clinicalised one, often ambiguous and confusing. It implies that if we stop 'active treatment' we in turn are giving up on the person, just leaving them to die without anyone doing anything to assist them. This couldn't be further from the truth. What it does mean in the terminal context is that where death is imminent and likely within hours or days, life sustaining, and life prolonging treatments will be substituted with comfort care measures which are maximised to better support the person receiving care.

Annette was supporting her dying mother. I'd come onto a late nursing shift and was informed Betty would likely die sometime throughout the night. Her three adult children were keeping vigil by her bedside. I was informed that family had requested 'active' treatment for Betty who was dying before them. I was confused about what was going on given the request to us was for full resuscitation the moment Betty died.

I went straight to Betty's bedside and could see it wouldn't be long. I spoke quietly with the family and asked them what their wishes for Betty were. As they sat by her side providing her with the love and comfort she required, there was a beautiful peacefulness surrounding Betty and I was mortified that at any moment I would need to destroy that. As things stood, when Betty died, I would have needed to ring for assistance and have the crash cart deployed. Betty's daughter, Annette, again confirmed to me they wanted 'active' treatment.

I quietly asked why they'd chosen active treatment and what their understanding of this was. Annette relayed a conversation with the doctor. He'd asked if they wanted active treatment for their mother and they'd replied, 'Yes'. I asked Annette her understanding of the term and what she thought it meant. She replied they believed we would do everything possible to keep Betty comfortable and not suffer any pain. I felt saddened in that moment knowing I didn't have time on my hands. The family wanted to say goodbye peacefully but had inadvertently agreed to the opposite.

When I explained what active treatment was, Annette and her brothers were understandably mortified. At any moment, when Betty went into cardiac arrest, we would be doing everything possible to bring her back. Annette immediately, and with a panicked look, said that wasn't what they wanted. I explained slowly and carefully that refusing active treatment meant we'd concentrate on keeping Betty comfortable and as pain free as possible. This would be our priority. They'd thought through the casual use of the term 'active treatment', with no explanation, that it meant we'd 'actively' keep her comfortable.

Following a quick midnight call to the doctor asking him to come back immediately to again have that conversation with family and to review the documentation, Annette, her brothers, and Betty were able to say goodbye within the peace of the moment, without any confusion or chaos.

The act of Compassionate care

There is a simplicity to Compassionate care and it's often in the simple things like the provision of dignity in care, the small gestures that have a power beyond compare. They come with a feel-good hormone that doesn't leave a nasty hangover. It's an all encompassing practice of good manners, showing respect even when rushed, and giving a warm smile and eye contact when speaking or assisting with a personal task. It's the continual reintroductions and lack of assumption that someone with dementia will remember a name or role. It's the extended hand to shake and connect with the person. It's showing a personal interest, by making light conversation about a person's life during a task or interaction. It's noticing details in someone's personal effects with genuine interest to show they're cared about.

Compassionate care is reminding oneself of what the person's been through, knowing their background, understanding the importance and significance of life events. It's about creating a version of the person's life, if their history is unknown, making it easier to relate to and connect with them. It is acknowledging the feelings of others, which can take but a moment, and show empathy by using sensitive statements such as, 'I understand'. If it's a difficult or frightening experience for the person, it's acknowledging this by a statement such as, 'I can see this has been difficult for you' or, 'I can only imagine how you're feeling'.

Compassionate care fits right where it's always quietly been, hidden alongside clinical and personal care. But by bringing Compassionate care to the forefront, together with clinical and personal care, they make the perfect trilogy. Together they bring a holistic care approach to those needing it most. Together they make magic happen. Compassionate care better equips a Dementia Doula to create an opportunity for bringing everyone together, including staff, to work together for better outcomes. It assists in taking away the unrealistic expectation that care staff, as individuals, can be everything to everyone and lighten that load bringing joy back into their practice.

Compassionate care fits in all the spaces that clinical and personal care can't reach. It's an approach that can fill in the blanks and also provide an opportunity to be more creative with care provision, a way to adapt to a unique or unfolding situation and be able to pivot when needed. Compassionate care provides a path for thinking outside of the box and coming up with new ideas to trial.

Leonie's story ...

I was working with Leonie and Martin. Martin was starting to show more advanced symptoms of dementia and the challenges for Leonie were beginning to increase. Leonie had hoped there was the possibility for one more interstate trip to visit friends together before Martin declined further. As the timing for the trip drew closer, Leonie became concerned that the instability that comes with travel would potentially be too overwhelming for Martin and he may at any stage respond in a way others may not understand. The responses of others would be pivotal in ensuring Martin felt calm and reassured throughout the journey.

Leonie contacted me with her concerns and wasn't sure what to do. We discussed the situation and what was concerning her most was Martin becoming upset and overwhelmed. She knew how this might play out for him and that others may see him as being angry and aggressive. If this occurred at an airport, security would likely become involved. Her fears were realistic. They needed a plan for moving forward. We explored the possibility of some individual handmade travel cards, that could be discreetly handed to staff or bystanders to give context for any events that may unfold.

On their return, Leonie shared that the trip had been rough on Martin. He'd struggled to stay connected to the everchanging environment and situation. She said that she'd used every single card I'd made for her and stressed the value she placed on each and every one of them. She shared the change in attitude in those around them when they took the moment to read the cards. These simple pieces of cardboard ensured everyone knew the role they played in bringing something to Martin when he was feeling lost. Leonie summed it up perfectly when she said, 'I would've paid $100 for each of those cards I handed out. That was the impact they'd had'.

Being creative with the care we provide doesn't have to be complicated or time consuming but creating a relationship and trust with our clients better places us for trialling ideas that may or may not work or may need adjusting. The importance is in the feeling of trust created with family members that we're prepared to provide support in any way we can. They're the perceived small things that can assist others to climb mountains and bring back a sense of normality to an otherwise complicated life.

Attributes for Compassionate care delivery:

To carry out and bring to life the role of the Dementia Doula, there are particular attributes that an individual will need to possess. These include the following:

Emotional intelligence: the ability to handle interpersonal connections with staff, those living with dementia and their families. It's having an awareness of one's own emotions and the emotions of others and working within this awareness. Knowing when and how to park one's emotions and responses and to 'read the room', picking up on unspoken words and feelings.

Resilience: having the capacity to reflect on things that happen while considering one's own personal values when working alongside the perspectives of others. Through ongoing self-reflection, a Dementia Doula can improve their resilience and that brings an increased sense of hope while reducing stress levels.

Critical thinking: the ability to think broadly and analytically and solve problems often without time on one's side. Critical thinking can influence creative thinking resulting in better outcomes for all and increased resident or client satisfaction.

Cultural awareness: keeping cultural considerations at the forefront of practice as they relate to an individual. This can influence a person with dementia's, and their family's, view of care provision and attitudes towards end-of-life care. It will also provide context for interpreting behavioural responses of the person.

Confidence: the ability of a Dementia Doula to communicate reliably and with conviction with a client, resident and/or family member, and represent their vision, along with that of the organisation they work for, about how both can function and move forward together respecting the position of each other.

Collectively these attributes support a Dementia Doula in creating an environment addressing that which is important to those they serve. The need for dignity, control and privacy is necessary not only for a good life but also a good death. Just because someone with dementia is unable to articulate these needs doesn't mean they're any less important to them.

When challenges arise, a Dementia Doula questions if something could be done differently and creates a theory of what that might look like. They consider how change could safely happen and what they could do to make it happen. They imagine an ideal world for people living with dementia and then use it as the blueprint. When the Compassionate care model comes to life, there's a flexibility that wasn't there before. If we can see it, we can create it, and make a tangible difference in this space.

Compassionate care supports ongoing change in a way never imagined. It creates a platform from which to challenge what's historically been deemed the norm, or accepted practice or how it 'should' be done. It shakes up thinking, challenges mindsets and opens possibilities for a different way forward. It has a power to reconnect relationships that appeared beyond repair. It prepares families for a role they never signed up for and a connection they never thought possible.

It's what we already do

There is a misconception within the health and aged care industry that Compassionate care concepts are already embedded into everyday practice. And while there's an intent to do so from those who care, there's often a lack of opportunity. A medical working shift is commonly filled to the brim with medical and personal care tasks and if there's a moment to spare, Compassionate care may get a look in. But it's unlikely to be care administered in isolation with no time allocated to the task.

Someone entering the world of the Dementia Doula from a medical background needs to ensure they don't bring a rigid and formalised skill set to the table. While such a skill set can create a strong foundation for the Dementia Doula role, it's important such attributes complement and contribute to Compassionate care practices, and don't become a substitute. There's no place for a hybrid version either - that's how Compassionate care gets pushed to the side. When working within a clinical setting, you're charged with fast paced sorting, solving and fixing, and while these are tasks a Dementia Doula also faces, they do so from a different perspective. Dementia Doulas add to this ever-changing landscape, allowing clients and families to just 'be' and assist in recognising appropriate timing for all.

Compassionate care in the Dementia Doula context doesn't always follow a script or run to a schedule. It's about being creative and at times making it up as you go along. It can change direction at a moment's notice and support a practitioner to provide reassurance, a hand to hold, a shoulder to cry on. Dementia Doulas assist when there is a pressure to fix. They are there when wobbly times come, to provide words of comfort and create clarity to move forward. A Dementia Doula is the person families first think of when a sense of hopelessness seeps in and no one else seems to get it or understand what appears like a helpless situation.

Compassionate care with a Dementia Doula

In a world always in a hurry, Compassionate care brings calmness to the chaos. It can slow down time to create moments where there's no urgency to get things done, fixed or managed, and avoid the trap of being influenced by a perceived crisis. When unwell or convalescing, the body automatically slows life down; it's often not a choice. The body needs rest and a calmness not found in the outside world. It often means temporarily retreating with a few days of tv, pyjamas and hot mug of tea!

Slowing down the chaos brings not only a sense of peace but an ability to reconnect without all the static. When working from a place of chaos, so many of the little things get missed - connections with others, the environment, the awe of nature, and those special moments along the way that can't be recreated.

Compassionate care is about being accountable for how every moment is spent, knowing those moments count to someone, knowing they can make a difference in the life of another. When you look at it and name it, you feel the power it truly contains. Within the health and aged care industry it's easy to fall into the trap of looking too high for where we can truly make a difference. This is the change Dementia Doulas bring. This is the change we can talk about. This is the change we can teach to others. It doesn't come with a perfect formula, or a how to guide. If it did, it wouldn't be called Compassionate care.

Compassionate care doesn't always go smoothly and may at times be met with resistance or heartache, but it still matters. It matters that we empathetically connect in a way that demonstrates to others that we've got their back, that we're there regardless and we see their pain. There may be bumps along the way that serve as important reminders for why Dementia Doulas are needed in the first place.

Compassionate care in the Dementia Doula context is diverse and difficult to frame. It may start with the formulation of a future plan, but it becomes about so much more. It is a focus on destigmatising and demystifying what lies ahead and tackling the complexities that accompany it. It's taking away the pressure of needing to fix and sort, and instead, to just let be. It was often the nightshifts, when things weren't quite so frantic, where I could just 'be' with a resident or patient, allowing them a chance to talk about fears, hopes and regrets. These times made me realise how different the opportunities were for someone dying from dementia: experience the loss of one's voice, to lose the opportunity to share and express the things that matter most to them with others. It was now time they had their chance.

Being frank, open, and honest and 'keeping it real', help define what everyone impacted by advancing dementia is experiencing and will ultimately face. It clearly identifies probable milestones, while empowering those involved in care to take a proactive and considered approach with the person with dementia's wishes when any interventions are considered.

Leaders in Compassionate Care

Dementia Doulas will continue moving forward as leaders in Compassionate care and do so with calmness and influence, walking the path with a 'can-do' attitude. Taking the 'can nots' and looking at them through a different lens, turning them into something that 'can be', having or initiating sometimes difficult and distressing conversations with clients and families when no one else will. And at times, a Dementia Doula may just be required for moral support, without the ongoing need for constant advice.

A Dementia Doula brings a confidence to stand up for the rights of others and to promote this by encouraging and engaging community ownership, connecting everyone so they all feel a responsibility for their neighbor, getting individuals to put up their hand and do their bit, especially when times are tough. A Dementia Doula is best placed to bring people together, even those with no idea what they have to give or what they could provide and inspires them to show up anyway.

A quality of the Dementia Doula role is in the additional skills and knowledge they often bring to their practice. It may be an additional interest or qualification in education, coaching, public speaking, counselling, psychology, pastoral care, writing life stories, and the list goes on. Weaving in the special extras means a Dementia Doula has so much more to give and a forum through which to share it and explore. I think of a Dementia Doula with counselling qualifications who can continue working extensively with the families she supports especially when issues of unresolved grief and loss or other traumatic events were to surface. Another Dementia Doula I know provides as part of her service, an opportunity to capture life stories so others will find it easier to connect with her clients. She offers this as an additional part of her service due to her skill set and training background.

Ultimately, it's a Dementia Doula that will lead families through the transitions they'll likely face. Life with dementia will bring changes from one day to the next and life as families know it will never again be the same. The life of perceived normality becomes one of constant uncertainty. Medical appointments and support services, packages, and funding, these become the terminology for where their future will likely head. For a Dementia Doula, it's about keeping the person with dementia front and centre, with families by their side, social networks encouraged and maintained, and families having somewhere to turn to. It's helping families to navigate the world of dementia by translating, summarising, and lightening the newfound load. The hope is in making the future just that bit brighter.

Preparing for the storm while the sun shines

For a Dementia Doula to maximise the client's experience, the optimal time for connecting is at the time of diagnosis. Individuals living with dementia will have unique experiences, but there are some likely milestones that are helpful for families to know about so the needs of the individual are catered for right from the start. This is also often a time of information overload for all involved and a time when a Dementia Doula can assist in deciphering the information provided along with the systems they're attempting to navigate. In doing so, families are better placed in their understanding of dementia, what's going on and absorb the information received.

At the time of diagnosis, along with all the information given, there's often a flurry of medical appointments, reviews, referrals, medications, brochures, care packages, assessments, and more. This is a time where relationships can be formed with the Dementia Doula for the long term, and a familiarity established with the person with dementia. It's a time to clarify the role of families and significant others. It allows families to continue being in the role they feel most comfortable, without the unnecessary burden of being defined as a 'carer'.

This is also the perfect time to get everyone on board, including the person with dementia should they choose, to put plans in place for a better tomorrow so they can all go back to living for today. With an uncertain future ahead, it's hard to enjoy the simple things in life while anticipating what's to come. This may include discussions about supported future care in the home or community and possible transitions into higher supported care. Dementia Doulas keep it real for families, giving them ownership and a sense of control, allowing them to steer their own ship and prepare them for situations before they occur.

A predictable path with unknown variables

The gift of connecting with a Dementia Doula early on is the gift of time, slowing down conversations and prioritising what's important to families in the moment. When families and clients feel overwhelmed, a starting point is not always obvious. By allowing a quiet space, without a sense of urgency, a Dementia Doula can help to bring perspective for all. Families and the person with dementia then have an opportunity to take a deep breath, take in what's happening and then go from there.

A Dementia Doula helps the family unit understand that they don't have to go it alone in navigating what's to come. They help give permission to slow things down and realise things can happen in their own time when they're ready. As important as well intended and funded services are, I still commonly hear families say, 'Please don't give me anymore help sheets or brochures, and don't send me to another website'. This is reflective of how overwhelming and distressing this time can be for families and the need to put the brakes on.

A carpark consultation

I remember driving a marked work vehicle once that clearly identified I worked for a dementia related organisation. As I headed back to the office one day, I stopped to grab lunch. As I got out of the vehicle, an older woman approached me and began telling me how her husband had dementia and how difficult it was for her. She spoke with sadness at how tired and exhausted she felt and the amount of care he needed her to provide. She was reluctant to leave him home alone while she went shopping but believed she had no choice.

This was a woman at the end of her tether. For whatever reason she hadn't been in a position to connect with services and wasn't sure what to do. Our brief carpark encounter was for her only intended to be an opportunity to share with someone what she was going through. I used this time to listen to her and validate the difficulties she faced on an ongoing basis. I commented on what an amazing job she was doing, keeping everything ticking along. I could see the desperation in her eyes even though she was asking for nothing. I could see she felt this was her issue to deal with as best she could.

I found a brochure in my bag and the last thing I wanted to do was overwhelm her. I opened it up and pointed to the bold phone number in large print inside. I told her I wanted her to call the number and tell the person answering the exact story she'd just told me. I shared with her there was support there waiting for her and all she had to do was ask. She took the brochure from me, took a deep breath, and let out a big sigh. I could see she didn't have the energy for more well-intentioned information, but begrudgingly started to read the brochure. I held out my hand to stop her and with a smile said, 'I don't want you to read the brochure, I just want you to call this number.' With that she took another breath, this time a sigh of relief. I didn't want her to have to think or process anything - all I wanted her to do was call. Support was out there waiting for her, but she had lacked someone to connect her to it.

Sharing the load and translating the information at hand is a component of Compassionate care that a Dementia Doula can offer, sometimes with instant results. The sigh of relief from this woman told me she knew then and there she was no longer on her own supporting her husband. It's all about timing. The right information at the right time and presented in the right way. If it's appropriate to give someone a brochure, clearly explain why they need that specific brochure in terms of the information relevant to them on that particular day and in that given moment.

Sometimes, like with the woman in the carpark, it's to simply share a phone number highlighted in bold print. If that's the case, ask nothing more of them than to just call the number. The amount of valuable information out there is fantastic but it's up to the Dementia Doula to sift through it all and bring out the relevant bits when appropriate and explain their reasoning behind it. It's unfair to put the burden on families, hoping they'll take all the information home and somehow sort it out for themselves.

Measurements of success

It's all well and good to find a way to be more creative and compassionate about dementia care, to make things happen in a different way, but how do we know we're meeting the mark, making a tangible difference that's of value to others? This is an area we must not show complacency in for we need to keep pushing ourselves to be better today than we were yesterday and to be better again tomorrow. Some key goals we will continue to strive for are:

- An increase in the number of clients being identified as being within the last 12-18 months of life
- A decrease in calls for ambulance services and hospital admissions
- An increase in the incidence of a palliative approach being initiated in a timelier manner
- Family carer satisfaction rates increasing due to the quality of information and support they've received
- Staff satisfaction rates increasing as they gain more confidence from education tailored to increasing their skills and knowledge and practical application of these for changed practice in end-of-life dementia care

Question for reflection ...

Could the practice of more formalised compassion-based care finally provide an opportunity for measurable outcomes?

The gift ...

An in-depth knowledge of dementia and its trajectory isn't necessary for delivering care with kindness, in a humane and compassionate way.

I hate watching people slip away and not having the chance to say goodbye ...

• Care Staff •

4 • Gaps that needed filling

'Advance Care Planning involving people with dementia and their families can provide opportunities to discuss and later, initiate timely palliative care.'

- Birchley et. al., 2019 p.825

As I looked into the eyes of families and those living with dementia, I saw they were desperate for answers, information, and something that made sense. They shared their lack of understanding and need for education to fully appreciate that which they were experiencing first hand. They knew they lacked opportunity to prepare for what was to come and were often stuck in the moment, just trying to get through today.

Without significant change in this area, families would continue to miss opportunities to play a more prominent role in supporting and caring for their loved one particularly during their final stage of life. By creating a new stand-alone role there would finally be a way to better service an existing gap for families and staff, to better inform them for decision making and planning processes and ensure comfort care measures were adequately in place.

Anne's story …

Anne and her husband John had been planning their future life together when things took a turn for the worst. John was diagnosed with younger onset dementia. Their world crumbled before them. I was given the opportunity to be one of the first contacts they'd had with dementia services. I will honestly say meeting them shook and saddened me. To meet with such a young couple facing this cruel disease together was something I struggled to comprehend.

Our first meeting together is still etched forever within my mind. The three of us sat together at their dining room table as I listened with sadness as to how John had, at the age of 52, finished working in his trade as a carpenter. I could hear and feel their disappointment knowing this diagnosis would significantly impact their future together, their dreams to build a house, their plans to travel. My sadness would turn to determination, knowing I needed to support them both in whatever way I could. I desperately wanted to bring a sense of normality back to their lives.

My role at the time provided an opportunity to connect and support them both but at the same time was limiting in what I could truly provide them. The gift for me at this point in my career was a planting of a seed that continued to grow over many years to come. I was grateful to have met a couple like John and Anne so early on, a couple who trusted me and shared with me their hopes and fears at a time when John could still articulate what he felt he wanted. He did this though, because of the program and service we, as a team, offered at that point in time. It was one that didn't offer sympathy and pity but one that extended the hand of friendship and offered guidance within the chaos they both faced.

They built a trust with our team and others in a similar position, and what we saw was John given the opportunity to connect with his new life, where he could share within a safe environment that didn't judge or finish his sentences. He had an opportunity to teach us about his experiences with early-stage, younger onset dementia in a way we never could have thought possible. As a couple, they gifted us with a view into their world and trusted we wouldn't change how we saw or treated them.

Catching up to the research

The Dementia Doula role is one responding to the shortfalls identified in current research, such as van Riet Paap et. al., (2015), which suggests that specialised end-of-life care in this area continues to be unequal or non-existent when compared with other life-limiting illnesses. The flow on effect means there are inconsistencies in the approach for building supportive networks around the person living with dementia to ensure their end-of-life plans are in place or enacted.

Crowther et. al., (2013), also supports what families were saying and experiencing, with their ongoing need to be included in care provision but feeling left behind. It had long been recommended that healthcare providers work more collaboratively to better meet individual needs and deliver appropriate care within a diverse range of care settings - a structured team approach that would place the person and their family at the forefront of care and be more responsive to those from culturally diverse backgrounds.

The Australian National Palliative Care Standards (2018) highlighted that people with dementia do require a different approach to palliative care due to the long unpredictable trajectory of the disease, issues in capacity for decision-making, communication difficulties and lack of the wider society's understanding of the disease. The standards reinforce how critical it is for people living with dementia and carers to be able to access high-quality responsive and respectful palliative care that addresses the individual needs of the person while still promoting quality of life.

Leading a coordinated approach

The Dementia Doula role provides support to those impacted by dementia at a time that for some, may be at their lowest point: they offer a beacon of light, and a hope that something can be done to make a difference, a hope that doesn't come with shallow promises or assurances that things will get better. Dementia Doulas demonstrate that power is in the preparation, formulating a plan well in advance, to be pulled out when needed or when the time is right, one that was compiled while the seas were still calm and thoughts more organised and structured.

When the hurdles seem insurmountable there's a need to instead adapt to the situation, do what we do best, one step at a time, rather than trying to fix the whole system. *Making moments matter* is the Dementia Doula mantra and that's what needs to happen. Rather than becoming overwhelmed with what's happening, we need to make moments matter, enabling our clients to take the scenic route and enjoy the sights along the way, acknowledging, and identifying what might be done in each moment they have rather than focus on what's been lost. We're still aiming for the peak, to get to the top, to make change happen for the person and their family, but we don't lose sight of the good things happening along the way. Let others concentrate on fixing the system at large. Dementia Doulas bring the focus back to the small things to be guided by and help others do the same - celebrate that smile, a restful expression, a gentle squeeze of the hand. Dementia Doulas start by acknowledging and celebrating the moments that often go unseen.

Preparing for the transitions

Transitions in life are often joyous occasions - the birth of a child, starting school, graduations, age milestones, weddings, and more babies on the way. Life concludes with a farewell through death. While not predictable in order, many go through these milestones in some way or another. When a diagnosis of dementia is received, transitions take on a whole new meaning and most are not welcomed or celebrated. Transitions continue to push a wedge through the normality of family life, bringing inevitable change for all, leaving wounds that sometimes never heal but always leave scars. Preparing for these transitions is essential, for it is during these times the losses may appear greater. Lack of acknowledgment and planning for these transitions by family units see them going it alone while at the mercy of well-intended service providers who steer families in directions that are not always best for their loved one.

Families immediately begin to pivot when they collectively discover their loved one has been diagnosed with a life limiting disease with no effective long-term treatment or cure. The odds or chances of someone with a diagnosis of cancer is different to that of one with dementia. They don't have an opportunity to share in any success stories with hope swiftly taken away. Dementia Doulas get to change what a success story in dementia looks like, how it can bring hope and play out differently. Dementia Doulas get to set a more positive tone, rather than a deeply saddened one. To ultimately achieve success stories that have more than one chapter, means moving the focus from all things medical and bringing what remains to the forefront, the person themselves.

Fears associated with the myths and stigma of dementia will exacerbate heightened emotions around the future not being what was thought it would or should be. There's a lot of information about dementia drawing eyes to the changing landscape, without an offer of any sense of control or hope. We can all fear something that hasn't yet and may never happen. It's important to gain clarity about some of these myths and this will only happen when talking to someone who knows and understands dementia in a holistic person-centred way.

Transitioning into care

After many a sleepless night, hoping for some type of relief, a new direction, a day that's better than today when those days never seem to come anymore, the term 'residential care' is bandied around to families. There are processes to follow, new services to navigate, meetings to be held, and what happens with the head isn't always followed by the heart. Where does the emotional processing find a place, or even begin? Families are told it's all for the best, it'll make life easier for all, it's what the person needs to keep them safe from harm. How does the person with dementia themselves, and their families, process this time, who do they now connect with?

As they face the possibility of residential care, there are limited opportunities to voice the sadness and loss families face, anger at difficult situations or the fear of control being taken away. Voices can become raised and family dynamics start shifting. Relationships at these times can be severed beyond repair or strained enough to make it difficult to come back from. With heightened expectations, disappointment and despair, angry comments are made, and vows broken. Who holds the family hand reassuring them they're not alone?

When entering into residential care, families enter a new system with new faces and constantly changing environments. This is the norm for those who work within the walls of a care home, but for those entering for the first time, it's a whole new universe. When peace and stability is needed, constant change leaves many struggling to find context or a comfortable fit. These changes can take away the voice of the individual overnight and their sense of place in the world. Changes can leave many feeling isolated, alone and in a world where care is simply accepted as how it should be.

Families enter the residential care world experiencing a range of emotions. It may be a time they felt they were prepared for, or it is the result of a decision made suddenly and quickly. Their emotions may be clearly defined or a mix of regret, sadness, guilt. They may even feel a sense of relief that their load is being lightened as their family member is finally receiving the care and support they need but are no longer able to provide.

Not to be underestimated is the continuing grief and loss experienced by the person with dementia as well as the family members involved. There may be a sense of losing the person and the guilt of feeling that there was no other choice but to put the person into care; that they've let them down, that they should have been able to step up and provide the level of care required, even though for whatever reason, it was no longer practicable.

Diane's story ...

Early on in my dementia career, I was asked to speak with a group of families all of whom were supporting someone with dementia within a specific care home. The brief as it was given to me had been that certain family members were being 'difficult'. The hope was to somehow get everyone on the same page. It was here I met Diane, wife of Paul, living with younger onset dementia. Because Paul was in his late 50's, he was still fit and agile. He had a strength that many others had lost with age. This meant that if Paul became upset, staff feared his physical responses were leaving them in danger.

I spoke with the group of family members for two hours and, during this time I was saddened to watch and hear of Diane's daily experiences. As I commenced the session, Diane's phone rang. She looked to me and apologised, she needed to take the call. But rather than leave the room she took the call in her seat. The rest of us could only listen. She naturally spoke with a strong voice but within it was a sound of frustration, despair with a twinge of annoyance. While she listened to the caller, her response was what shocked me. Diane replied with, 'I'm already here, I'm here, I already am. I'm in that talk in the next room. I'll be out shortly.' Diane's call ended. She was now unsettled, and I took a moment to check she was okay. She shook her head and shared that these were the calls she received from staff numerous times a day.

Diane would assist her husband with lunch every day and given it was 11.30am, staff were wondering where she was. The fact she was already there appeared lost to them; they needed her assistance and they wanted it then and there. Whenever Diane's husband showed signs of becoming uptight, staff would call Diane, day or night, to make the trip in to calm him down for them. My jaw dropped. Not only was I mortified Diane was paying for care she was inadvertently delivering herself, but I couldn't help but wonder who was out there supporting the staff. How was Diane going to have any type of relationship with her husband when her sole purpose was putting out spot fires?

Transitioning into new types of relationships

Relationships undoubtedly change and become more difficult to navigate with dementia. A partnership where two became one may now again become two. Relationships, solid from years of work, constant negotiation, sacrifice, sharing the good and the bad, navigating life together and the challenges thrown their way, begin to crumble. Dementia leaves no plan for how to put relationships back together. Instead, people can feel shattered into pieces too small to be fixed.

How do families redefine their relationships or work out where they now fit in the bigger picture? Do they just grab a new seat? Dementia can see children become parents and partners become carers. Families take on a new dynamic as roles shift sideways. The person with dementia, known as the rock and stability of a family unit, now becomes the person who requires nurturing, no longer the 'go-to' for advice, understanding, or to get out of a jam.

They are navigating the wedding vows, the promise to never give up, through sickness and in health, a vow that perhaps should have an allowance to include others helping in times of sickness, the inclusion of a plan A and a plan B. Instead, this sense of obligation and love can leave a partner feeling as if they can no longer fulfil their side of the deal, that they're letting their partner down. What a burden for one to carry and carry on their own! Who provides them with an opportunity and breathing space to talk through their place in all of this? Who supports them with the emotional weight they often carry silently hidden away in their heart?

Due to the pace at which this transition often occurs, and the practical decisions that need urgent attention, these feelings and emotions are likely to go unnoticed. They're unlikely to be recognised, with little time for them to surface, or be acknowledged or any assistance given. What the world may see from the outside is a partner who is snappy and impatient, one struggling to let go of control, one that's probably going to be a problem moving forward.

We all need to do better in this space and the Dementia Doula role was created with this very scenario in mind. If these challenges aren't identified for all involved with the chance to offer real assistance, then families will continue to navigate this time alone, with no clear leader and with no one that can read the map. The battle is all but lost before it's even begun.

Transitioning through lack of opportunity

When you step into the mainstream palliative care world, one accessible to anyone without dementia, you see processes and systems in place, purpose-built units and hospices aimed at providing specialised comfort care for people at their end stage of life. But for someone living with dementia, there is currently nothing specific or tailored. There may be an ad hoc approach in place where the term, 'palliative care', is bandied around, but there is still the lack of a clear plan or direction for someone with dementia. Someone living with dementia simply isn't eligible to be even considered for hospice services in spite of dementia being life limiting. How a dying person doesn't fit the criteria for hospice care doesn't make any sense!

A service without a contingency

I recently spoke with an Oncology Registered Nurse working within community-based cancer treatment and support services about the eligibility criteria for what they offered. I wanted to check whether access to services was an anomaly only within the area of higher care or something starting much earlier. With sadness, she shared how frustrating it was having a patient referred to their service with cancer, but if it was discovered they also had dementia they were automatically excluded from the program and service. How is that fair AND where is someone with dementia supposed to go then?

In their study, Swerissen and Duckett (2014), reveal 60-70% of Australians expressed a preference to die at home. It highlighted that statistically only 14% are able to achieve this. With dying so highly institutionalised, moving away from this medicalised model in the final stages of dying is harder now than ever. To die is a normal part of living and historically dying occurred more often within the community setting. This provided those within one's own community the opportunity to either provide support to families during the dying phase or connect more easily with them, to pay respects when the person died and to then support those grieving.

Too many terms create confusion

There is commonly an inconsistency in the use of the terms 'palliative care', 'palliative approach' and 'end-of-life care' with terms often used interchangeably.

Palliative care is the care provided to someone when they are advanced in their disease and actively progressing with little or no chance of a cure. They're expected to die, with the priority being to optimise quality of life, comfort care and treating symptoms as they arise. A holistic approach would be in place ensuring all aspects of care are considered and include the person's physical, emotional, spiritual, and social wellbeing.

The choosing of palliative care will often be influenced by multiple factors, not just personal preference of location. Considerations still need to be made for the person's condition, amount of care required and whether constant care is available to provide the necessary support.

Principles of palliative care are affirming of life, regarding dying as a normal process. It doesn't purport to either hasten or postpone death but instead focuses on providing relief from pain and other distressing symptoms, while integrating all psychological and spiritual aspects of care. The primary goal of palliative care is to put support systems in place assisting someone to live as actively as possible until death, and to help families cope during the person's illness and bereavement.

Palliative approach focuses on improving and enhancing quality of life for someone with a life-limiting illness and their family. It doesn't assume that death is imminent but continues to provide comfort and relief of symptoms throughout the condition's trajectory. It involves focussing on early identification and treatment of pain and other issues with consideration for physical, psychosocial and spiritual aspects of care.

The benefit of a palliative approach is the ability to implement it at any time during the disease or illness progression. It provides the opportunity to move away from treatments intended to "fix or cure" and focuses on maximising comfort measures.

End-of-life care is initiated within the last few weeks of someone's life, as they rapidly approach death. Their care needs are likely to be higher during this time. It's during this period where an increase of palliative care services and support are required, ensuring comfort measures are maximised with family feeling supported. It's care delivered when death is imminent and will extend into bereavement care for families and possibly staff. Such care provision would be coordinated and delivered by a specialised health care team.

Not everyone's on the same page

In practice, this may mean palliative care wishes are not discussed until end-of-life is imminent e.g., within hours to days. There is a need for greater understanding of terms not just for families but also for staff. To be able to clearly differentiate between the three terms opens the door for earlier discussion and planning to take place for staff and family. A clearer understanding of these terms used within the palliative sphere will better position everyone involved in identifying what the main goals and expectations will be to support the person with dementia. To know the priorities of such care will be firmly focussed on providing comfort, support, warmth, and security to better meet the person's needs will be reassuring to families and assist them in accepting what is to come.

With palliative care and dementia finally becoming a natural combination, the Dementia Doula role is best placed to influence the aged care sector moving forward to address the individual and specific needs of people and families living with advancing dementia. Dementia Doulas continue to speak to those like Pearl and her husband by keeping the most basic element of the need for kindness at the forefront. Dementia Doulas assist in defining a palliative care approach within the dementia context, one continuing to strengthen confidence in moving away from mainstream generalised care provision to one with a focus on a definitive outcome for those with dementia.

A focus of a Dementia Doula is not in the doing but ensuring the provision of comfort care measures rather than active life prolonging treatments. They don't support euthanasia for someone with dementia, but rather support a good death. Dementia Doulas ensure clients have a choice and enable those living with dementia to receive palliative care in a manner that reflects dignity and is inclusive of existing Advance Care Plans. This is a role that creates an opportunity to influence the well-being of the person through environmental considerations and appropriate tailored comfort care.

A common misunderstanding

When I first started using the term 'palliative approach' many years ago, I remember being challenged. I reflect back to discussing with care home staff about how beneficial a palliative approach could be for someone living with dementia and on one particular occasion, was met with strong and angry responses. I was challenged that implementing such an approach meant I was, 'Just wanting to end someone's life sooner'. The more I tried to explain the true meaning of a palliative approach, the louder the voices got. This wasn't an isolated case and it saddened me that the system and those in it weren't yet ready to openly discuss another way of thinking, especially when it came to better supporting someone with a life-limiting condition.

Today I feel comfortable having such a conversation about a palliative approach to care for people living with dementia. There's more receptiveness to palliative concepts and its benefits. The challenge now is normalising it in everyday practice. It never was and never will be in the same realm as euthanasia. There are no similarities. Comparing them highlights the damage that could be caused, and the confusion created when open and honest conversations don't happen. I don't suggest they're easy conversations to have, but they at least get everyone on the same page. What we can't and shouldn't assume is all medical and care staff will know all there is to know about palliative care, how a palliative approach could be integrated into care and how this fits within the complexities of dementia.

It's not fair to think those without palliative care skills or training would be able to identify someone requiring a palliative care approach. Dementia Doulas are best placed to initiate these conversations and to work alongside staff and health professionals to get everyone onboard. Families must continue to be included in these conversations with sensitivity, as many will be filled with fear. Their knowledge base should not be assumed. They will also likely need assistance with their understanding of such terms and how they fit into the bigger picture for their loved one.

Question for reflection ...

Why do you think it would be important to discuss your wishes with those closest to you?

The gift ...

Palliative care for one should be palliative care for all.

Death is but a moment in time but dying is something we can truly influence

• *Dementia Doula* •

5 • Snapshot of a better day

'Every individual will have a different idea about what would constitute 'a good death' for them. This may include being treated with dignity and respect, being without pain and other symptoms, being in familiar surroundings and being in the company of close family and friends.'

- Mitchell et. al., 2016, p.55

Preparing for a better day is to first understand and see what that might look like. In making a difference to the lives of others, a Dementia Doula must have a clear understanding of what they, as the support provider, is wanting to achieve, ensuring the proposition is realistic and practical. With that in mind, a Dementia Doula shouldn't become discouraged when others say something isn't possible or can't be done. The impact of taking a step in a different direction can be huge when a clear goal is in sight and strived for. Making a difference can come in the most unassuming ways.

A Dementia Doula recognises they can't be an island, knowing they can't physically and emotionally be everything to everybody, and that by doing their bit as part of a professional health team they become a vital cog in an ever-spinning wheel. Ultimately the Dementia Doula is best placed to support not only families and direct care staff but also to provide a pathway for referral from Aged Care Specialists and General Practitioners, giving them an option for offering a continuity to their service by advising their patients of a further support avenue available to them encompassing Compassionate care.

The following story highlights the significance of connecting with others passionate about making a difference.

Meredith's story …

Meredith was an aged care volunteer I'd met years ago. As part of the volunteer program, she'd been buddied with Doris. Doris resided within the high care memory support unit of a care home and Meredith would spend time with her throughout the week. She would share activities, crafts, conversations, and both enjoyed walks in the garden together. Over time, Meredith had a feeling something wasn't right. She'd spent enough time with Doris to realise she perhaps wasn't where she should physically be residing. Meredith knew Doris had a diagnosis of dementia, but she never appeared too advanced in the disease. Doris spoke about wanting to leave with an ability to communicate and connect which was surprisingly advanced for someone in high care.

It took time for Meredith to flag her concerns. She was after all, 'just a volunteer'. Her nagging feeling wouldn't go, and she eventually reported her concerns to someone she thought might listen. Her feedback was taken on board with Doris being reassessed. It was discovered Meredith's insights were correct, and Doris was relocated to a low care part of the home where she had the freedom and independence she'd so longed for. Because of Meredith's insight and her confidence to report, along with her connection with Doris, Doris's quality of life was changed for the better. Her sense of well-being increased, and she reconnected with a life she'd previously known. When we come together to truly share the care, it's amazing what can be achieved.

Down the dark void and beyond

A Dementia Doula recognises the inevitable losses a person living with dementia faces and plays a significant role in planning and preparing for these times. They strive to minimise the carnage caused by dementia and better prepare families for tomorrow. Dementia Doulas continue to bring a sense of hope when all seems lost, with the aim of preparing families for visiting loved ones in supported care, connecting in positive and meaningful ways they couldn't have imagined, finding a sense of peace that while dementia has taken so much, it hasn't taken everything.

Creating better days for all

Preparing for a better day isn't just about families, it includes the person living with dementia, the staff along the way and, of course, the Dementia Doula themselves. It's about collectively nurturing and supporting anyone impacted by dementia in a way not seen before. It's an opportunity to think about what aspects a Dementia Doula can influence today, tomorrow and for the long term, to frame what a better day could look like for all impacted by advancing dementia. Let's explore the new benchmarks we're collectively aiming for, the changes that need to be made, and reflect on how they could be achieved.

A better day for those living with dementia is ...

An open line of communication acknowledging the personhood and humanity of the person living with dementia provides a better day. Being part of honest conversations delivered with sensitivity and compassion, brings hope and opportunities to take back control instead of seeing it diminish. These conversations aren't always easy for someone living with dementia, but their impact can be life changing.

When someone with dementia has the chance to be heard, there's a collective understanding. By taking away unnecessary pressure and unrealistic expectations, everyone involved can start from the same page. When someone with dementia makes their views and position known, and feels respected, there's a better chance for more fluid decision making taking away any doubt.

Those living with dementia need to be assisted in navigating their feelings of grief and loss, a process that may be explored alone or together or a combination of both. More than ever, it's important to keep connections alive through empathetic listening and sharing of thoughts. Being included in conversations can be helpful for both the person with dementia and their loved ones. It provides the opportunity to share feelings about living with a diagnosis of dementia, how it impacts their inner self, and their everyday experience of life. In return, being open to the shared experiences of those who love them most can also be beneficial to the person with dementia.

A better day will include a person living with dementia being better placed and supported in making and contributing to their own planning, formulating their own questions, and providing input for future care prospects. They are better positioned for interviewing prospective care homes well in advance of the actual time of need and having a say about where they believe they'll likely feel best supported. By fostering relationships earlier, a Dementia Doula is better placed to create and encourage better opportunities for those living with dementia to be included more in decision-making processes.

When someone with dementia is supported in this process early enough in the disease trajectory, they develop a better understanding that forward planning will ultimately decrease the chances of suffering, discomfort, or discontent later down the track. They are better able to know that their input will alleviate or minimise future uncomfortable or awkward situations and distressing conversations for family members. They can feel empowered knowing they've played a part in ensuring their family are on the same page in understanding what their wishes are. They can feel relieved in knowing that they planned so their family didn't have to guess.

A better day will be the opportunity to live within an all-encompassing care environment where the person feels safe and nurtured; within a calm setting with excess noise reduced, a trusted space that truly feels like home, where there's a larger room available when death is imminent, to accommodate family members and those wishing to stay overnight or for extended periods of time, a place where cultural and spiritual considerations previously captured and clearly documented are incorporated into their care.

- A better day for someone with dementia brings respect, humility, inclusion –

A better day for families is …

Families need to feel supported as they enter the higher care world with a bundle of emotions and unknown expectations. It's a foreign land often different to anything many have ever experienced, and with it comes a new language, different ways of thinking, new systems, routines, and smells. Unless families have previously supported someone with dementia, they've no idea how to play the game, how to respond or to react, what to ask for, how they need to be. A Dementia Doula is best placed for guiding this process for families and providing that much needed clarity.

A better day is showing families that all is not lost, but often well hidden behind the wall of dementia. By moving forward together we create a more cohesive relationship, an open line of communication to decrease the risk of any misinterpretations, where requests and intentions are understood, and false hope alleviated.

A better day is finding a middle ground where quality of life exists not just for the person with dementia, but for families as well, finding the good on the darkest of days, where it would be easier to just give up, finding the positives in times when all appears lost. A better day is looking to tomorrow with renewed passion for what could be achieved when expectations match the reality. It is preparing for whatever is coming and knowing that the best laid plans must come with an adaptable and flexible mindset, bringing everyone together to meet a common goal, to forge a new path in an unchartered terrain.

A better day for families is feeling supported by a Dementia Doula, being taught how to love and connect again, to be a family once more, to come together as a united force. It is to hear and be guided by the person with dementia, to feel they're not alone, to know those around them care but are often not sure how to show it. It is to be guided in how to include those wanting to play their part, allowing others to share the load and know what's needed from them. By taking families back to the basics, where true clarity can begin, Dementia Doulas support them to be better positioned to experience and share bottled up emotions that fill an unprepared heart. For families, emotions can surface quite suddenly and without warning, and contain feelings of regret, sadness, guilt as well as relief that the person is finally receiving the care and support they're no longer able to provide. The Dementia Doula can support families on their emotional rollercoaster.

A better day for families is having a feeling of security, knowing Advance Care Directives are completed and in place, and if not, being guided by a Dementia Doula in the creation of one. A directive brought together and based on the person and their life story, without feeling pressured to get it perfect or right, helps families feel comfort in having made a start on their loved one's wishes. Peace can be knowing that all those that surround their loved one are doing everything possible to support but not hasten, a peaceful and comfortable death within the final stage. A palliative approach ticks all the sought-after boxes and supports life with no intention of shortening or lengthening it. An approach allowing the person to just be in a state of comfort and peace while still being connected to those that matter.

- A better day for families brings hope, connection, honesty -

A better day for staff is ...

A better day for staff is learning how to truly connect with those they support, to have the opportunity to share in care with compassion. Staff passionate about dementia care can finally have their own voice and influence how end stage dementia care could and should look and be better recognised for the vital role they play. It is developing a better understanding of palliative care and a palliative approach and how it fits into their practice. It is feeling more comfortable in identifying when a palliative approach should be initiated and how they should go about doing so. Building staff confidence, knowing they can develop the skill set needed to ensure residents aren't sent to hospital unnecessarily, which ultimately creates confusion and distress for the person with dementia and unnecessarily fills up acute care beds.

A better day for staff is knowing that specialised palliative care training would better support their professional and personal growth and better equip them in changing what care could look like for someone living with advancing dementia. It is feeling more confident about end-of-life care and the role they could ultimately play. Knowing they had easy access to specialised palliative care services would enable better care for the person with dementia.

A better day for staff is having the opportunity to contribute in a way that allows them to be the best version of themselves, to be part of a care environment that helps them to nurture and build on the qualities and strengths they already possess. It better positions them to be a significant part of change in palliative care and assists them with seeing a new way forward for dementia care. It allows them to develop an environment where they can be more creative in the way they respond and be more inclusive. To be more committed to embracing the challenges faced by culturally and linguistically diverse (CALD) communities, those experiencing homelessness, lesbian, gay, bisexual, transgender, queer, and intersex (LGBTQI) communities, post-traumatic stress disorder

(PTSD), and veterans. It is knowing they make a tangible difference.

A better day for staff is feeling heard and acknowledged for what they want to be able to provide for their residents and for what they already do. It is to work in a rewarding workplace where everyone has common goals in how to optimise good care, one that supports staff retention through better recognition of the challenging role they play.

- A better day for staff brings recognition, inspiration, motivation -

A better day for a Dementia Doula is ...

Dementia Doulas thrive on having ongoing opportunities for personal and professional development. To have the opportunity to stay connected to a supportive Dementia Doula community allows them to share in the wins and losses, along with highs and lows. They create a role for themselves that connects with their sense of purpose, knowing they fill existing gaps and can be responsive to the needs of families in a timely manner. Dementia Doulas provide a way to build trust and form relationships with families that can set them up for the challenges that lie ahead.

A better day for a day for a Dementia Doula is having a plan ready for when the time comes. It is an ability to stay connected with families assisting them to be a part of a more coordinated approach, one that ensures others hear the voices of the person with dementia and their family. It's being better positioned to help families with the creation of a plan B, for when plan A doesn't necessarily work out. Dementia Doulas ensure they continue finding the positives, the wins when hearts are breaking, to celebrate new connections and the forming of bonds, tapping into that which remains hidden. A better day is bringing it all together in a way that all makes sense to those involved.

- A better day for a Dementia Doula brings relationship, creativity, strength -

Brenda's story …

A few years ago, I conducted an information session for families supporting a loved one in a high care dementia unit. 30 people sat before me waiting for some understanding of what they were tackling. The session was highly emotive, and I could see many tears being shed. One particular woman caught my eye. Sitting right at the back, she cried for the two-hour duration and approached me individually at the end. Still emotional, her words ran deep. Brenda, the daughter of a resident said, 'Thank you, you've given me hope.' I was taken aback. In reality, all I'd given the group collectively was two hours of my time. I'd spoken honestly and sincerely. I'd not promised a cure or a better tomorrow, yet still she'd used the word 'hope'.

Brenda then shared, 'I nearly didn't come tonight, I'm just so tired of hearing the same things over and over. I was ready to give up on my dad but now you've given me hope.' She described how down it made her feel continuing to hear the same information on how she should support her father and how she should go about doing it. She was spent. She was ready to give up. She was broken. The look of guilt in her teary eyes was a defining moment for me. It was in that moment I realised I'd shifted from being a Dementia educator, to being a Dementia Doula.

Brenda went on to say she had a newfound understanding of what her dad was experiencing, how every moment of every day was an unrelenting struggle for him. She now saw her dad from a different perspective. She knew it wasn't going to be easy, but she'd put the pieces of the puzzle together for herself and could now see the new role she could play in supporting her father.

This connection with Brenda had a profound effect on me. This turning point gave me a snapshot into a world that was possible. If this had proven to be a way to connect in such a short amount of time, what could an independent role such as the Dementia Doula achieve when given more time and an established relationship-based connection. Things for me were starting to make a lot more sense.

Question for reflection …

What could a better day in dementia look like without any limitations?

The gift …

The prospect of a better day can fill others with a sense of hope for a better tomorrow.

I spend so much time on the things I have to do that I rarely get an opportunity to do what I really want and need to do …

• *Care Staff* •

6 • The weight of grief and loss

*'It is critical that people living with dementia and carers
are able to access high-quality palliative care that is
responsive, respectful, and culturally appropriate.'*

- Palliative Care Australia & Dementia Australia 2018

When working with family members supporting someone with
dementia, there is often an experience of long term, continual
grief and loss. Helping families to navigate this time is not as
straight forward as it may appear. The complexities of grief
often change a person's normal response to everyday situations
and at times can risk relationships with others. Knowing when
and how to connect families to broader support can be a vital
step for moving forward and can also be important when the
bereavement phase is reached.

Anne's story continued …

*I think of Anne from chapter 4, who went on for many years
alone and feeling emotionally shattered until the day John died.
I attended John's funeral and could feel the tangible love that*

surrounded Anne on that day from those of us wanting to share in her pain. I stood saddened that I hadn't done more for her and John. That the collective band of love should turn up today was significant. But Anne, had been saying goodbye to John for the previous 6 years and, in many ways, this was just another day of farewells. This realisation shook me in a way I couldn't have imagined.

Four years later, I reconnected with Anne for lunch and was saddened to see her grief was as raw that day as it had been on the day of John's funeral. Anne had heard the well-meaning comments that John was now in a better place, he was no longer suffering and that she could now move on. But Anne wasn't in a better place. She was continuing to suffer, and she was far from ready to move on. While she knew the words to be true, she tucked these well-meaning statements into her heart alongside the pain that had never been acknowledged or treated. She'd locked up that part of her and put back on the beautiful smile she was known to carry. The pain inside would continue to grow.

Catching up with her was humbling for me, as she opened up that box of pain, hidden away from public view, and shared it with me for the short time we had together. What I saw was an outpouring of grief as though John had died last week or even last month. Anne was trapped within her own life with a part so broken still wedged firmly within her heart. She never wanted to forget John, she did want to move on but, sadly, had no idea how to go about it.

For Anne, and so many others facing continual loss and lack of direction because of dementia, the lack of recognition or acknowledgement of grief and loss within the dementia context is very real and brings a misunderstanding and disconnection. For many family members this is often a hidden burden they carry. Families, and the person with dementia, often suffer in silence with the roll-on effect seen as heightened emotions or absence of family members or a reduction in visits. All this ultimately impacts on the wellbeing of the person living with dementia and has a capacity to drive wedges within families. The 'system' lets the Anne's of the world down in a way we can't imagine. The physical needs of the person with dementia are met as they present, but the depth of the emotional pain we don't see goes untreated and unacknowledged.

The problem with grief and loss is the societal perception of who is most likely to experience it. There's a misconception that grief and loss is experienced by the loss of someone through death, rather than as a natural response to any significant loss. It can be experienced at the same level of severity following the breakdown of a relationship, the loss of a pet, a job or even a way of life, or the loss of a previously good health status which is something often experienced by a person given a diagnosis of dementia.

Navigating the emotional changes

Dementia leaves many lost and confused, disillusioned and broken. It leaves many feeling as if life, as they've known it, will never again be the same. While there are still moments of laughter, joy and happiness shared, families are often too exhausted to fully appreciate those precious moments. The Dementia Doula assists families in pressing 'pause' on their lives to see things how they really are, allowing families to acknowledge, in a safe space, that life is pretty challenging at times. They help acknowledge that dementia has impacted them in as many ways as it has the person themselves. Families need guidance in recognising and owning that they aren't on the outside looking in. They're very much part of the experience.

For many this leaves feelings of guilt, or that their loss isn't as great as the person with dementia.

Acknowledging the realness of feelings is the starting point for moving forward. Dementia Doulas can't fix these feelings but can help clients feel comfortable with their raw emotions. Feelings should be validated and, should they get in the way or take over in a way that's not productive, then it's not a sign of weakness to seek professional help. The following provides useful suggestions for connecting with clients. They are conversation starters for risk factors possibly contributing to feelings that may be experienced by clients as emotions spill over and uncharacteristic responses may be seen. By doing so, a client may not only receive much needed support but also be better placed to be treated for undiagnosed depression or underlying anxiety issues.

According to Beyond Blue in Australia, factors increasing an older person's risk for anxiety or depression include:

- pain
- increase in health problems/conditions
  (e.g., heart disease, stroke, Alzheimer's disease)
- side-effects from medications
- losses: relationships, independence, work and income, self-worth, mobility and flexibility
- social isolation
- significant change in living arrangements
  (e.g., move from independent living to care)
- admission to hospital
- particular anniversaries and memories they evoke

(Beyond Blue – Risk factors for older people, 2022)

When reviewing this list, it's easy to see the risk factors apply to both the person with dementia as well as their family members. While family members often go it alone without personal support, many of those diagnosed with dementia miss out too. It's easy for responses and reactions of someone with dementia to be put down to their condition without a review or treatment plan in place for anxiety or depression, let alone grief and loss.

Dementia Doulas assist in navigating the incomprehensible, a life turned upside down causing chaos no one could have imagined. A dementia diagnosis instantly strips away a person's being and takes away plans, hopes, and dreams for the future and leaves behind a palpable sadness. Dementia Doulas are in a privileged position of being able to be with people during their time of ongoing loss, on their darkest days. For families and the person with dementia, this will often be one of the most difficult and challenging times of their lives.

The losses in dementia turn the life of not only the person upside down but there's a roll-on effect to anyone connected to them. The losses experienced through a diagnosis of dementia will be influenced by many different elements and will all impact on how a person with dementia and their family grieves. Even within a family unit the experiences for all involved will be different and, as unique individuals, they will react accordingly. A person's culture, their upbringing, religious influences, beliefs and previous experiences, will impact their grieving process.

The definition of grief from the Oxford Dictionary is:

a deep or intense sorrow or mourning. It is also described as *mental suffering or distress over a loss, sharp sorrow and 'painful regret'.*

Grief and depression are different but can have similar characteristics. Both can lead to feelings of intense sadness, insomnia, poor appetite and weight loss. If changes experienced by the individual appear to impact on the way they interact within relationships or live day-to-day, then it's important the Dementia Doula recommends they get further support or professional help. Grief is an emotional response to loss. While it could be due to the loss of a relationship, moving home, change in health status, divorce, or death.

If someone close develops dementia, the losses may appear in a differing form. Families are faced with the loss of the person as they were, the loss of the relationship previously shared, along with plans for the future. While grief is an individual feeling and experienced differently at different times, in the context of dementia it doesn't always become easier with the passing of time because the person is still very much alive.

By understanding the grieving process, Dementia Doulas are better placed to assist those going through it and to provide connection in a non-judgemental manner at a time when others may not be best placed to do so. Grief will affect every part of a person's life, their emotions, thoughts and behaviour, their beliefs, physical health and sense of self. It will impact on their identity and relationships with others. Grief can leave those we support feeling sad, angry, anxious, shocked, regretful, relieved, overwhelmed, isolated, irritable or numb. While grief has no set pattern, everyone will experience it differently. Given the long trajectory of dementia, the experience for many may last for years. What a Dementia Doulas does is validate these feelings and work with families to acknowledge them and seek professional assistance if required.

Dementia Doulas aren't experts in grief management but should still be aware of the signs. It's not the role of a Dementia Doula to fix a person's grief, yet it is useful to understand some of the patterns and traits that may be experienced in order to best support families throughout these losses. By understanding the complexities that go with grief: denial, anger, sadness, heartbreak, guilt, despair or loss of hope, acceptance and love, Dementia Doulas are better able to connect with families.

While grief is an area highlighted due to the impact it has on families, it must be recognised when the emotions of others tap into or trigger a Dementia Doula's own feelings. While being involved in the grief of others, this experience may bring up feelings of fear or previously experienced losses of the Dementia Doula. If there have been similar experiences of loss, trauma, or guilt, these can rise to the surface bringing back painful feelings and memories. The Dementia Doula must not only be sensitive towards the family, but also be aware of one's own feelings in order to manage them as well. Personal support plans should also be in place for the Dementia Doula to ensure that when connecting with families, personal issues aren't shared and don't impact conversations.

Dementia is unique in as much as it creates an unusual situation for families. The person with dementia gradually leaves their loved ones while still being very much alive. Families 'lose' the person long before their physical death occurs.

Anticipatory grief and dementia

Anticipatory grief is not talked about in this area and not commonly recognised as part of the process family members may experience when supporting someone with dementia. Families will often express feelings of sadness and hopelessness at any time following a diagnosis of dementia. It's common for families to experience grief even before their loved one has died, and it may happen at any point during the progression of the person's dementia. Families are unlikely to identify with it as an experience of grief and loss, even though the feelings and emotions experienced are similar in nature to a loss experienced through death.

Anticipatory grief may happen within families when:

- the relationship with the person with dementia starts to change
- thinking about how dementia might impact the person in future
- it's more difficult to remember the person they once were
- the person with dementia becomes more withdrawn from family events and conversations
- the person is no longer physically or mentally present with other family members
- considering the loss of future plans together

A Dementia Doula can reassure families anticipatory grief is not a reflection on them, that it doesn't mean they're giving up on the person or love them any less. Families will, early in the dementia journey, start thinking about the impact dementia will have on their future lives together hence the term 'anticipatory grief'. There's a risk of getting too far ahead too soon, the risk of a perceived sense of urgency in making certain decisions. Preparing families to acknowledge that while the feelings they may experience can be just as intense as an actual bereavement, it doesn't mean they'll feel it any more or less following the death of the person.

Facing the time of bereavement

Everyone will react and cope differently following the death of their family member and will react to bereavement in their own personal way. Many people will go through grief without needing professional bereavement support. How family feel and respond after the person has died may be impacted by different things which could include:

- their relationship with the person
- previous/past experiences with death
- individual personalities of family members
- how they've responded to changes while they were caring for the person
- how much they've already grieved throughout the progression of the dementia
- the circumstances surrounding the person's death

There may be a range of emotions experienced by families after the person has died, some of which may even be positive. These feelings can include:

- shock and pain (even if the death was expected)
- sadness
- anger and resentment about the person's experience
- guilt or anger about how the person was cared for
- emptiness or numbness, as though feelings are frozen
- being unable to accept the situation
- feeling isolated and a lack of purpose
- relief, both for the person with dementia and themselves that the physical suffering is over

Because the person being supported would likely have lived away from the family home over many years, it may be difficult for families to process the fact that the person has gone. This may result in 'delayed grief', where it takes someone longer to accept the person has died. It could also be due to the feelings at the time of death being too overwhelming to deal with, or many practical things needing arranging, or other things going on in their lives. All may leave little time to grieve.

Delayed grief may happen for a family member if they've cared for the person over a long period of time and possibly leave an emptiness for family members as they experience yet another role change. A family member suddenly losing their carer role may find themselves with additional free time, having possibly disconnected from hobbies or interests over the years. Social connections would also likely have changed and the disconnection from a former life may become more apparent. This has the potential for family members to experience feelings of loneliness and isolation as they adjust to a life without their loved one in it.

Accidental counsellor

Dementia Doulas often find themselves taking on the role of accidental counsellor. These are times where we share in difficult conversations with our clients, whether they're someone living with dementia, their families, staff or even the wider community. The support role we play means we often respond to their pain and suffering. While not usually qualified in formal counselling and/or identifying as offering counselling that doesn't prevent us from being in a position where those we support share with us their pain, sadness, and suffering. It's not about asking us to fix but to just show up, to listen and be present.

To see families stuck in grief is something that can leave us feeling as if we're unable to do our jobs properly. To see families struggling is a sadness we carry knowing the strength of our role is in standing by them throughout the progression of dementia, continuing to provide an opportunity for them to talk, to vent and to be heard, to hear them express feelings for someone who died years ago but feeling as if it was just last week. A Dementia Doula's privileged role provides that touchpoint for families, to normalise that which brings the greatest pain so that those impacted by dementia never need feel they're going it alone.

The power of the truth

By taking the lead with truth telling, the Dementia Doula can make life easier for families and caregivers by alleviating the possibility they will at some later stage be put on the spot, in situations they may find confronting or difficult. Knowing the truth earlier can reduce the chances of awkward and difficult conversations being had when emotions are heightened. Without honesty, the end of someone's life may be difficult to accept, with it appearing as if from nowhere as a surprise. With honesty, there's unlimited opportunity to share thoughts and feelings and to begin processing emotions long before the time comes.

Truth telling within dementia care can be difficult to navigate. What is clear in this area is when the truth is withheld or an untruth told, it can leave feelings of deception that are difficult to come back from and re-establish trust. Even when well-intended, the result is often more harm done than good. Telling the truth to the person with dementia and their family can be difficult. It is hard to hear things that create pain and sadness, but if it's done with sensitivity and from a place of compassion, this can ultimately build a solid relationship based on trust for moving forward together as a united front, where no one's left behind.

While being honest can be challenging and at times difficult, it can also be empowering. While it may stir up a range of emotions and feelings for the person with dementia, families may be better positioned to understand, process, and know what they're dealing with if it is done in the earlier stages of a dementia diagnosis. If any of us are excluded from conversations to save our feelings or alleviate sadness, we tend to make up our own stories regardless of what's going on. We still try to make sense of a situation. Sometimes these stories are bigger and more distressing than navigating the truth itself.

By being honest and sensitive there is more chance of building trust with those impacted by dementia and them knowing who they can rely on and who will give them an accurate version of what's going on, even if it's something they don't want to hear. Truth telling is a way of creating that safe space for a person where they can express feelings and know they are being heard. It has the capacity to give back a sense of control, even if there appears to be no hope. It prevents the possibility of unnecessary anguish or sadness and can take away the burden of making difficult decisions. It can make what appears overwhelming, more simplified when put in an understandable context.

Advocacy – being the voice of reason and representation

A strength of the Dementia Doula role is being an advocate to those they serve, to be the voice for those who can no longer speak and represent themselves, to say what would be said if the situation was different and the person with dementia could speak for themselves, or families felt more strength and confidence. A Dementia Doula is aware of their motivation and position when speaking on behalf of others, ensuring they represent the views and perspective of those involved and knowing they should avoid using opportunities to share information as a platform for personal opinions or grievances.

The advocacy voice a Dementia Doula uses must come from a place of persistence and not from frustration or anger, for if that's the case, the messaging to staff, family members and others, risks being blurred and altogether lost, as those on the receiving end become defensive and shut down.

True advocacy in the dementia context is about keeping things on the agenda, being persistent, remaining vigilant. I learnt this skill from my son when he was younger. He worked out quickly that demanding and yelling wouldn't get him anywhere and he taught himself persistence. Calmly and quietly, he would ask, 'But why can't I? But why can't I? But why can't I?' until achieving the desired effect. It's a great skill to have. It can wear down the strongest of minds and greatest resisters and all you're required to do is just show up and keep talking calmly and with conviction. The reality is, if we don't speak on behalf of our clients, who will? Who will be their voice? If it's not us, or families, others will have no choice but to make it up as they go along.

A Dementia Doula then is best placed to ensure services and care provision are more accessible and readily available for someone living with dementia, which is currently not the case. They'll ensure this access flows into areas not traditionally utilised within the dementia context and include palliative care services. This would ultimately benefit areas that may include but are not limited to – culturally and linguistically diverse (CALD) peoples, regional & remote communities, Aboriginal and Torres Strait Islanders (ATSI), returned services people with post-traumatic stress disorder (PTSD), the homeless and those exiting the prison system.

Shared voices …

Being a voice for those living with dementia is about stepping into any opportunity that presents itself. A few years ago, I spoke at a forum to 100 community members about supporting someone with dementia. I knew the audience would be made up of predominately family members supporting someone living with dementia. I felt it important to acknowledge the constant and unrelenting role they played at times with little to no support. I thought about the stories I'd shared with families and those living with dementia over the years and the messages they'd wanted others to hear and understand, messages they felt unable to convey themselves. It was in that moment, I realised this wasn't an opportunity to say what I thought people wanted to hear, it was a time to say what needed to be said, to share messages I'd been entrusted with and to bring them to life in a way others could connect with.

I continued asking myself what those living with dementia would want to say if they'd had the opportunity and confidence to speak to the audience that day? What messages would they share that would assist others in making their lives just that bit easier, smoother? I proudly represented those I'd worked with over the years and others I hadn't identified in the audience. I shared the stories and perspectives of dementia entrusted to me. I spoke with a passionate voice ensuring no one missed the messaging. I could see tears amongst the crowd. I wanted all who listened to not just hear the messages but to feel them too, to connect in a way they perhaps weren't expecting. I cared so much about their experience too.

I knew they wanted to do more, were likely searching for answers to the many questions they had. I'd worked with families who couldn't grasp dementia as a concept. They still saw the person they knew, the one they'd lived with for many years, and they weren't sick or unwell. They were just being 'stubborn', they just wouldn't 'step up'. They 'refused to meet anyone halfway'. These were the comments I'd heard over the years, and these were the misconceptions about dementia I wanted to address in a way they would hopefully understand.

I watched as the group nodded in acknowledgment of what I was saying, giving examples of where we as support providers often get it wrong. At the end of the presentation, I was met with a queue of people all wanting to share that they now saw things differently. They realised they were setting their expectations too high, that the person they loved could no longer reach the benchmark previously set or even make meaningful sense of it.

The voice I'd used was mine, but the words belonged to those I'd met along the way. They also belonged to the many others out there living with dementia. In that moment I chose to use words entrusted to me, to speak on behalf of another. As Dementia Doulas we'll likely have many opportunities in many different settings to advocate for those we know, but also for those we'll never personally meet or even know their name. The advocacy role sits much larger than just the person before us and it's up to us to take any opportunity that comes our way.

Question for reflection …

Are we really expecting staff within the aged care industry to have specialised skill sets in every aspect of health and aged care? Is that not realistically unattainable?

The gift …

Grief isn't just for a moment, it's something with the capacity to last a lifetime.

She (nurse) needs to get back to work, listening is the job of the social workers, not us, we don't have time for that stuff …'

• Hospital Nurse •

7 • Preparing for a better tomorrow

'... that efforts to improve QoL (quality of life) might focus on supporting relationships, social engagement and everyday functioning, addressing poor physical and mental health, and ensuring high-quality care.'

-   Martyr et. al., 2018, p.2137

Our greatest gift to families is not only preparing them for what's to come but also bringing them back to today, focussing on connection, turning them into one of our most utilised and valuable resources. We can flip things around and better position families in knowing what they have to give. We can help people with dementia to transition from living in the community to moving into care and we can help others to connect with their family member. Awe inspiring families already step up and do an amazing job and do so with very little guidance and support. They somehow manage to cope and adapt; so, imagine what they could achieve if they knew what they were doing in a way they could better connect with, rather than someone else 'stepping in and taking over'.

Missed opportunities

At the first ever family session I conducted, I was ready to share information with family members about what was to come with regard to dementia. I was speaking to a group of families supporting someone in higher care. They already came with a lived experience of dementia. I prepared myself for the complex and difficult questions I thought I'd be hit with. I was floored by the very first question. A family member asked, 'Can you tell us the difference between dementia and Alzheimer's disease?' I stood there in disbelief and felt sad and deflated. This was a question that should have been addressed at the point of diagnosis and it was coming from families many years down the track.

These families had supported their loved one for up to 10 years in the community and yet they didn't even know what they'd been diagnosed with. The system had let this family, and others like them, down. They'd navigated those years at home with little understanding or guidance about what they were facing, without a proper name for a disease they could look up, and yet they somehow managed to cope and do what needed to be done.

I made a conscious effort in the years ahead, to ask families what diagnosis their loved one had, and I continued to hear uncertainty or at best a guess. This wouldn't happen with any other condition, but families do what families do and that's take it on the chin. They do their best in a situation that's challenging and often without a confirmed diagnosis. This is where a Dementia Doula can support and educate and create a better understanding earlier and be that ongoing resource. They don't have to have all the answers, but they'll certainly know where to find them.

For me the obvious starting point for change was in bringing someone's personhood and their humanity to life, so that others could better see who they still truly were at the core, giving them a voice at a time when they were at their weakest and most vulnerable. A Dementia Doula can connect families to the medical and care world so that they are better placed to advocate for the person, to pick up on signs of pain, discomfort, hunger, thirst, a need for touch and a need for quiet. They can become more aware of subtle signs and changes and be better placed to identify them. They can be more empowered in the whole process and become the true voice of the person.

There are ways we can support this process and guide others to do the same. Within the family's own personal community network, there will likely be those who bring strength and ongoing support. The Dementia Doula plays a role in supporting those individuals to become as involved as they wish to be. Often support networks move away early on when someone is diagnosed with dementia, not because they don't care, but because they're not sure what to say or do. Dementia Doulas guide by assuring these significant others that their love and support will have an impact they'll never fully appreciate. A Dementia Doula may offer them useful tips such as:

- Never be afraid to ask the person or the family how they're feeling. Each day is different for someone who's grieving and experiencing dementia, so encourage them to take the time to listen and understand what the person is going through.
- Continue to talk about everyday life, with the losses experienced not always needing to be discussed or referred to.
- Ask the family directly what they could specifically do for them.

A Dementia Doula will continue to work with families in the ongoing building of their community of support. This community might be composed of family, friends, neighbours, church members and even the person's health care team. It includes anyone wanting to offer their support in some way but just not sure what to say or how to go about it. If the person with dementia has played a significant role in the lives of others, this inclusive approach provides an avenue through which others have the opportunity to give back and say thank you. This structured aspect of the Dementia Doula role captures what others wish to offer and how this could likely be facilitated.

Thinking and being creative

Preparing for a better day is about not aiming too high. It's being realistic about what can be achieved and staying in the moment with someone, reading their tone of voice, their body language, hearing what they're trying to say and what they need from us, getting creative with what could be done to ultimately change an outcome for the better. It's about asking what needs to be done to make it happen. It's having a vision of what a better day might look like, then working to make it come to life one way or another.

When you feel no one understands …

As a paramedic I was once tasked to assist an unwell woman named Ivy who was living with dementia. She was firmly refusing to go to hospital and had no interest in speaking or engaging with us. At face value she appeared scared and frightened, alone and feeling ganged up on. She knew no one was on her side. To her, all we wanted to do was just take her away. What Ivy needed was an ally, someone she felt was on her side, and who she felt understood what she was going through. She needed someone to see her as the person she was and not just a job number on a case card sheet. It didn't matter how much we comforted her and explained what was happening, she wasn't haven't any part of it and she wasn't going anywhere.

I moved away and let my partner do the talking, to give them space. I looked around her room and spotted a walking stick in the corner. I proceeded to pick it up and danced with it like I was in some musical stage show. I did it because there wasn't much else I could do. I didn't want Ivy to feel I was just standing there staring at her. While she watched my impromptu and very average performance, Ivy looked at my partner, rolled her eyes and asked, 'Is she for real?' and he replied with, 'I'm afraid so'. Instantly they had a connection.

My self-pride and ego were big enough to take the hit, to be the one they could both look at, roll their eyes, and connect. They both thought I was an idiot! I smiled internally with a satisfaction of knowing I was unlikely to make any sort of connection with Ivy, but in that moment, where the spotlight was taken off her, I watched how she now looked at and spoke to my partner. I knew she finally felt safe.

Understanding what's going on

Sensory changes are a known part of dementia and will be experienced in different ways by different people. This aspect alone changes the direction of care from generalised to custom built. Exploring some of the known changes possibly experienced, means everything done for someone with dementia should be carried out with caution and adapted if any distress or discomfort is noted. The brain is like a computer, processing the information that's been entered into it. The senses are designed as a type of information gathering system, sending messages to the brain for interpretation. With damage to the brain tissue, it's likely those messages will become muddled at times.

The following are examples of changes that may impact care provision and connection:

Hearing – Hearing may become impaired with someone finding it difficult to interpret what a sound is, or the direction from which it's coming. It may be difficult for someone with dementia to process sounds especially when there is more than one happening at the same time, for example, people talking while a television is on.

Smell – Hallucinations or olfactory smells can misguide the brain into thinking there's a smell of smoke or other unusual smell, where no such smell exists. This may cause alarm and unnecessary stress for someone with dementia.

Taste – Taste can be altered with it being suggested that chemical type tastes can taint food and alter an eating and dining experience.

Touch – The sensation of touch can become altered, with an increased sensitivity to the skin. The lightest of pressure may cause a pain sensation which may also be described as burning, hot or irritating.

Sight – If the occipital region of the brain is damaged, this can affect vision. If we think of the eyes in simple terms such as a camera, the eyes take a 'photo' of a setting or object and send that 'photo' to the back of the brain for processing. If that 'photo' is of a mobile phone, the brain may confuse the image and identify it as a block of chocolate. It would then make sense if the person then started chewing on it.

With physical damage occurring to the brain cells, interpreting messages through sensory input becomes a lot more complicated and confusing. This is an instance where the responses from those around the person become pivotal in how things will likely progress from that point. If someone is told off for chewing on a mobile phone while thinking it's chocolate, or there's an attempt to take the phone from the person, they're understandably going to get upset and respond accordingly.

Finding one's safe space

Part of the Dementia Doula role is assisting families and the person themselves to find and/or create their own personal safe space, a physical or emotional area where they can come to just be themselves. It's a space that's trusted without judgement or pressure. It's not forced, but a space where you as a Dementia Doula either invite others in or they invite you to join them, a space where it literally feels like time is standing still and the world outside no longer exists. It's where someone can invite others to join them, to walk alongside them rather than pushing or pulling them in a particular direction.

Creating or identifying safe spaces will be different for individuals. This space may assist those within it to seek clarity for decisions that need to be made or a best path to take. It gives the person an opportunity to feel comfortable exploring the options they may or may not want included in their future care. It may assist the person to tap into or reconnect with a spiritual side they can draw upon to find peace within the noise of the outside world or allow reflection on where they've come from and what that means for today.

When a safe space is created, it's easier for people to tap into their true feelings and to slow down the world around them. It becomes a place without expectation, a place to just be, to take stock of the situation. Confusion may become clarity through the quietness in order to navigate the unknown, to see a clearer path when unsure what to do, to not feel rushed. The space can be anywhere. It may be a physical place, a person or an object, something that brings with it a sense of comfort and reassurance, a moment to catch one's breath: a walk in the park or on a beach, to sit by a lake, a room full of cushions, a vegetable patch, a tinkering shed, a comfy chair on a verandah, a glass of wine with a friend, no rules, no expectations, time spent asking nothing in return.

Harry's story …

A few years ago, I had an opportunity, to perform a living wake. A friend contacted me on a significant anniversary of her parents that was to occur as her father lay dying in hospital with advanced cancer. It was the day of the anniversary and at 11am my friend contacted me to see if we could, 'pull something together'. By 3pm we had a script, decorations, a new dress for her mother, someone to play requested music on a guitar AND, the special part with such short notice, 20+ people standing in the foyer waiting to cram into the small hospital room and then spill out into the corridor.

The joy in Harry's face was palpable, with tears flowing freely from those of us surrounding him. It felt so natural, so normal, that we would come together to celebrate this anniversary and a life well lived. As the ceremony was ending, accompanied by the quietly strumming guitar, 20+ of us softly sang 'What a wonderful world'. As we concluded, 20+ friends and family instinctively formed a line and held Harry's hand while speaking their final words to him. There wasn't any awkwardness in what to say. They just spoke from their hearts and then left. As I approached Harry with my final goodbye, he smiled from ear to ear and with the little energy he had said, 'I don't need a funeral now.' This should be what a normal experience is for all, including someone with dementia.

A trusted presence

To be a trusted presence is an absolute gift to give another. The Dementia Doula has the honour of often being a trusted presence who provides the ability to slow down time and be a way to connect and be present for the caregiver, the person with dementia or for both. Sometimes just being there and saying nothing can give others unwritten or unspoken permission to just be themselves, to take away the pressure of feeling there are things that should be done or that need to be fixed and to just be in the moment.

It's the ability to be a presence that encourages others to trust their own intuition, to go with what feels right. Dementia Doulas create an emotional space where everyone feels safe and supported enough to follow their wishes regardless of the opinions of others, knowing that even if they change their mind or things don't go to plan everything's still ok. They help families to feel it's important just 'being there' rather than getting everything right.

As a presence, Dementia Doulas have an opportunity to see behind the scenes. They witness the rawness of what families face and are better placed to meet them where they're at. A Dementia Doula is able to find and access suitable support that are required in the moment. In order to share the burden carried by families, a Dementia Doula must first be trusted with the contents. It's then that answers may be found to the questions families didn't realise they had, or to problems they'd felt helpless to fix.

Sophia's story ...

Sophia was living with advanced dementia within a care home and was finding it increasingly difficult to settle at night for sleep. Care staff tried different approaches but nothing they did seemed to make a difference. Through a new set of eyes, Sophia's history was revisited revealing a strong religious faith that she had practised throughout her life. This important information hadn't been incorporated into Sophia's care plan and had fallen by the way. It was identified that Sophia's spiritual needs were unlikely being met. As her dementia continued to decline, it was possible Sophia was finding it more and more difficult to initiate staying connected to her faith.

A recommendation was made to purchase a set of rosary beads which family had confirmed she'd once owned but had lost. A card was printed with The Lord's Prayer and placed in her bedside cabinet. It was recommended that staff, while settling Sophia, hand her the rosary beads, sit with her and read The Lord's Prayer from the card so she could join in or connect within the moment as she needed. By acknowledging the significance of this for Sophia and providing her with an opportunity to reconnect with her religious faith, meant she was able to settle more easily in the evening.

Use of language

Reviewing the language used by those surrounding someone with dementia is important for where that language places them in the bigger picture: whether it's useful or considered, productive or obstructive and whether it brings out the best picture of the person we represent. A Dementia Doula should be aware of the role they play in modelling language that's respectful and to speak in a way understood by all. An awareness of language and references being used by all involved, provides another avenue for influencing culture change.

Dementia Doulas may assist families with the reframing of dialogue they may be using with a family member, and within the environment they reside. By listening to what we say and how we say it, what we hear around us, all sets a tone for how others will perceive and view dementia and the person experiencing it. It will shape the thoughts and feelings of others.

Many of us have had the conversation about what we do for a living. When we say, 'I work with people living with dementia', the reply is often, 'Oh, how sad'. But do we find it sad? As with any health care job, there are aspects that are sad, but also many that aren't. We share in the sadness and challenges, but also the joy and happiness, the connections, the celebrations. For many of us it's the most rewarding job we've done. It's not sad when you see someone looking relaxed and comfortable, when a special moment is shared, or faces light up when a child or pet enters the room. These are the stories we should share with anyone within our own communities to remove the assumption everything about dementia is 'sad'.

Language has the power to set the tone of any conversation. If we say working with people with dementia is sad, it creates a barrier that many will not want or fear to cross. It says to others that visiting someone with dementia leaves you feeling sad, and no one wants that. We know that's not always the case. We can change and influence the perception of others and how they feel, by continuously reviewing whether terminology and words we use are appropriate.

When used effectively, language can empower. Language should be respectful to those it refers to. It should promote a sense of optimism, peace, and dignity. Language can create and build a sense of connection. It can change how others see the person living with dementia as an individual, bringing back their sense of self, showing staff and families who they still are. Language can do the same for staff, valuing their practices rather than just focussing on what they've missed or haven't completed.

Language plays an important role in raising awareness and promoting dementia to the wider community. It can help to reduce the sense of fear experienced by many encountering dementia. Those with lived experience of a parent or a grandparent with dementia are often touched in some way, with no real understanding of it. There is an unrealistic fear of contracting it themselves or of not knowing what to say or how to respond to someone with dementia, scared of an unpredictable outburst. These words create an unnecessary fear, creating walls that lock someone with dementia in, almost like a smear campaign against dementia where the person is ultimately punished.

Whether through casual conversation or a formal presentation, language sets the tone for understanding dementia and the person experiencing it. Educational opportunities are ours as Dementia Doulas, to create a positive perception of dementia. We do this in the way we speak and respond to others, what we accept and what we correct. A common term used by news media is, 'the dementia sufferer', yet not everyone with dementia 'suffers' or if they do, it may be a moment in time like for all of us and not a label we would want to carry. If it's perceived someone is always 'suffering', it influences how those around them will speak and act towards them.

Language is a powerful tool and correct use of language and terminology should be included in the Dementia Doula's toolkit as well as that of anyone connected to dementia care. Correct language doesn't require additional time or resources. It can be utilised and implemented easily and has the power to move mountains and change a landscape. It can inform and create hope.

Marlene's story ...

Marlene had been a nursing sister during the war and worked overseas. While Marlene never spoke of these times, as a registered nurse in training I was fascinated by the job she'd done during the years she served her country. Marlene had dementia. She was blind. She was immobile. Her preference was to spend her days in her room listening to the radio. Beside Marlene's bed, on her side table, was a beautiful A4 portrait of her young self in her military nursing uniform.

What I was to reflect on many years later was the connection staff had to her. I think back to the way all staff approached her, how they spoke to her, the conversations that were shared, and I remember the joy of being assigned to her care. I asked myself why this experience with Marlene had been so different to that of interactions with other residents, why the body language and tone of voice of staff changed when they entered her room, then it clicked for me.

I realised we as staff hadn't been conversing with Marlene with dementia, but with Sister Marlene, someone we could connect with, someone whose world we shared. We knew she outranked us and deserved all the respect in the world, and while she wouldn't share her war stories, we filled in the missing pieces as best we could and created a life for her that helped us as staff connect with who she really was. We spoke to her in a tone that reassured her we could still see her, and I think of the medications she was given with the nurse explaining to her what they were for, assuming she knew what was being referred to. We spoke to the portrait, the photo beside her bed that brought her to life for us. It didn't matter whether she understood or not, she was made to feel part of the team. She was treated as if she was on staff and was supported as such.

Bringing Compassionate care to life

Compassionate care challenges a Dementia Doula to consider what they do and can offer in this space, to think about those things they've done on autopilot and those moments they've consciously thought about influencing. Compassionate care creates moments that value add to a person's experience, treasured special moments they can now tuck away for a rainy day. A Dementia Doula may not change the whole world of dementia, but they will change the world for an individual. They will start conversations, continue those conversations, and keep the conversations at the forefront. They will walk alongside families while challenging the mindsets of others. They forge a path for a better way of thinking and a smoother one for moving forward.

These moments can be simple and uncomplicated, like a compliment on an item of clothing or hairstyle, or the offer to change a tyre. Whatever it may be, it counts and has the power to change the course of someone's day. We may never hear the outcomes or the thankyou, but as Dementia Doulas, we smile knowing they're out there. Practising genuinely on others can not only build one's confidence but can often open up opportunities that would have otherwise just passed on by.

Picnic for Audrey ...

Audrey was a regular hospital patient of mine, being treated for a chronic health condition. Her family lived interstate and she was always on her own. I grew fond of Audrey. Even through adversity she continued to smile and crack a joke, even when it was evident she was suffering or in pain. In passing, we'd chat and laugh about a picnic we'd one day go on and what that might look like. As her health continued to deteriorate, and her hospital admissions became more frequent, the day came where I realised we had left our run too late. There was never going to be opportunity for that picnic.

I spoke with a nursing colleague about this, and on a day off, we decided to pack a picnic basket and take the picnic to her. A carefully placed tablecloth, a little imagination, and her hospital bed became the picnic setting. Audrey's face lit up with a grin from ear to ear. She struggled determinedly to straighten up in bed. She nibbled on food I knew she had no hunger or energy for. She enjoyed her picnic, shared stories and crumbs were inadvertently left behind. I never thought I'd seen her happier which highlighted how close the end was for her. My colleague and I spoke the words she was at times too breathless and weak to speak. We enjoyed just a moment in time with Audrey, but the memory has stayed with me over the years.

Audrey died a few days later. Family hadn't made it in time to see her or be by her side. What I hoped was that in some small way we had given her a deserving send off, knowing she was loved, appreciated and admired, not just by her family but by those she had infected with her beautiful smile. While it hadn't been in our job description, we'd brought some sunshine to her final days. We were there only to meet her care needs and treat her symptoms but going outside those parameters felt more natural and genuine than any drug we'd administered. It felt like a complete fit for the role we should be playing. We knew there was a line, and it was one we never crossed. Audrey was still our patient, but not acknowledging the connection we'd formed over the years would be to dismiss the essence of what we do - to care. We did care, we knew how to care, and care was what we'd delivered until the end.

Question for reflection …

Can we change the perception of dementia and remove stigma just by bringing a sense of normality to the lives of those who live it?

The gift …

Innovative approaches to improving dementia care means the sky is the limit for what can be achieved.

I have tears in my eyes at the prospect of this new venture (Dementia Doula role) and knowing the difference it will make. If only Dan (husband) had that understanding and right to be heard in his final stages.

• Wife of husband with dementia •

8 • Building a collaborative community

'Practising compassion requires a facilitating social architecture promoting norms of trust, concern and empathy, in which compassion is treated as a collective responsibility.'

- Bivins, Tierney, Seers, 2017, p.1025

By strengthening the networks surrounding someone with dementia and tapping into the diverse skill sets, we are better placed to strengthen the support the individual living with dementia ultimately receives. Working *with* families, instead of *for* them, results in a winning formula ensuring everyone's load is lighter and the experience is more rewarding. A Dementia Doula has, as their priority, the person and their family, but clinical and care staff also fall within their scope. Staff historically do their best every day, trying to be everything to everybody while knowing, as well intentioned they may be, it's just not physically possible. By creating a better and more productive connection between families and staff, Dementia Doulas enhance learning for all and form a solid team approach where everyone feels better supported.

Obstacles encountered

Another identified challenge experienced by many working within the industry, is the difficulty in meeting the needs of someone with dementia when the person can't verbally share what they want or need, particularly if the services of a Dementia Doula were not engaged until later in the disease progression. A lot of assumptions will be made on the person's behalf, and this highlights that listening to the unspoken messages they communicate, reflecting on previous wishes and more comprehensive conversations with family will continue to be the best care indicators.

Working alongside families with differing internal dynamics will always bring challenges. Some family members will want to contribute more than others, and some will be struggling to express or acknowledge the grief and loss they're experiencing. It is evident this will be a time of high emotion for all involved and will likely continue over a long period of time.

Sharing the care

A core value of the Dementia Doula role is relationship building, which is essential for creating strong links between themselves, families, staff, community and ultimately the person with dementia. The uniqueness of the role is in fostering the intuitive and instinctive approaches demonstrated by individuals and creating a more formalised approach which not only offers consistency of practice but is one that can be easily replicated.

By creating a community of care around the person with dementia, a Dementia Doula brings together a uniform and consistent approach, enhancing and maximising collaborative opportunities. It utilises skills of all those who surround the person, tapping into their expertise, where all contributions find a valuable fit. From the health care professionals, and families, to care staff and a neighbour, anyone willing can be included in this dynamic team.

Sharing care with health professionals

A Dementia Doula is best placed in supporting, General Practitioners, Aged Care Specialists and other health professionals by providing a continuity of care to them and their patients. Instead of feeling there's nothing more they can do, they can refer on to the services of a Dementia Doula when medical options are exhausted or there's a need for psychosocial support to be offered in tandem. A more holistic approach gives health professionals more options to share the care and support them in their ongoing connections with the person and family.

By recommending Compassionate care as part of ongoing care, the dialogue starts earlier allowing for a future with more tailored treatments and comfort care opportunities. The Dementia Doula gives health professionals somewhere to go. It doesn't leave families hanging or feeling they've been deserted. Hospital admissions are often unnecessary and stressful for someone living with dementia, and a costly intervention to the health system. They're often a last resort for staff and are the result of a lack of conversation, plan or palliative approach in place to ensure comfort measures are maximised and staff are briefed on the roll-out with families informed and included in the decision-making process.

It wasn't uncommon in my paramedic days to be called out at 2am in the middle of winter to pick up a resident with dementia from a care home. We would take them to hospital, away from their warm and familiar environment because staff hadn't identified the person was dying or were unsure why they were so uncomfortable. I was saddened by the frightened, confused expressions on their faces and would offer comfort, knowing it fell short. This unnecessary disruption would be confirmed three hours later when we were called to take the resident back home again, all due to a lack of understanding by caring staff, with no clear plan in place for what to do and with no involvement from families.

If someone with dementia is unwell or distressed, decisions will often be made quickly; staff don't always have time on their side to think through their responses. There's often a common assumption that conversations about a course of action, should a specific scenario present itself, has already been had. Sadly, too often they haven't, or the Advance Care Directive is hidden away in case notes, not readily accessible. If a conversation has been had it's not always in a legible form to be handed over quickly and easily to the next care provider that comes their way.

Sharing care with care staff

When working with care staff, it's vital for a Dementia Doula to demonstrate strong leadership skills and qualities to gain confidence and inspire desired change in others - change that staff willingly sign up for because they see a better path, not because they were directed to do so. A Dementia Doula is then best placed to support care staff in their ongoing understanding of dementia as a life limiting disease from time of diagnosis.

They can help inform staff that those with dementia will, in the future, be more likely to come with a plan for how they want their wishes to play out. Staff will be a pivotal part of a person's care and Dementia Doulas can help and support them in the role. By assisting staff with their understanding of dementia, and the significance of a timely tailored plan, the need to find different and new ways for supporting someone with dementia becomes more evident. This will include a clearer vision for navigating the disease and earlier identification of the terminal phase of the condition, and in turn empower staff in implementing an approach they feel comfortable and connected with.

The Dementia Doula, in working alongside care staff, can help alleviate feelings of burnout and stress. These known stresses are often the result of:

- lack of support, including lack of opportunities to talk about distress
- lack of knowledge about residents
- inability to interpret or meet residents' needs even when known
- feelings of powerlessness within care environment hierarchy not feeling listened to or taken into consideration overwhelming feelings of responsibility in difficult situations
- frustrated desire to make lives better for residents

(Edberg, Bird, Richards et. al., 2008)

Without the support of a Dementia Doula, staff will continue with generalised care provision and lack the necessary skills for identifying that a person has entered the palliation stage. They will continue to lack growth in a role they could ultimately find more rewarding. The Dementia Doula is better placed to support staff to see the value of more tailored comfort measures that don't necessarily require more time and resources but more a change in thought process.

Dementia Doulas should, where possible, be a united front with care staff who recognise they have the potential to ultimately become as much a voice for someone and their family as Dementia Doulas are. Care staff are a vital link to the physical care environment and to family. Dementia Doulas can assist in bringing care together in a way care staff may not have previously thought possible. When staff are gifted an opportunity to see a resident's life through a different lens, they begin finding their own answers and begin to ask more questions. When staff are better connected to the life story of those they serve, they instinctively begin tailoring their approach to better suit the individual before them. When they personally feel the difficult and traumatic stories of those with dementia, they're better placed to become who the person needs them to be.

A Dementia Doula can better inform the practices of care staff by creating an awareness of the instinctive and intuitive aspects they often already bring to dementia care provision. They put the spotlight on the challenges people living with dementia face and the worth of standing up for the person as an individual. When staff are more aware that they as an individual, can change the course of someone's day and experience, everyone's world has the potential for becoming that bit brighter.

Sharing care with families

By sharing care with families, a Dementia Doula is able to utilise a commonly untapped resource. It's within families that information for making today a better one is held, stored, closely guarded, and contains gems that will support the person with dementia. They often hold the key that service providers are searching for. A Dementia Doula supports families in taking an element of ownership over care provision, to be able to direct care in ways that better connect with the person.

Rather than the existing practice of taking care away from families, the Dementia Doula is in a position to give it back, adapting their role into one that suits family lifestyles. Family members have historically been underutilised, and we desperately need them as part of the team. In the current climate of a short-staffed care industry, it's more important now than ever to get them firmly onboard.

Families are often unaware of the gems they hold about caring for their loved one with dementia and need training and guidance for recognising the power they possess. They need insight into the strength of the role they could play and the differences they might make. They need to be nurtured into becoming a stronger voice in holistic care provision and it's exciting that a Dementia Doula can be an integral part of that awakening.

A Dementia Doula can assist family members in creating their own role, one that brings purpose and meaning even to the shortest of visits. To change the routine for families, those that often feel like they're just going through the motions of looking at the clock, knowing what day it is, making the trek to the care home, to go through the same routine they went through yesterday and the one they'll do tomorrow. It doesn't matter if they're visiting every day, once a week, once a month or even once every six months, it's the quality of those visits that counts rather than the number. Everyone has a vital role to play.

When a role is more structured and expectations better framed, families have more scope and become more creative in what the possibilities could be in supporting their loved one with dementia. What they contribute and how they do it becomes clear. It may even renew connection, especially when visiting can at times feel like a scripted chore. Clear expectations have capacity to reinvigorate families through giving them a new sense of purpose and structure to feel comfortable in visiting more often and taking on a more active and rewarding care role.

Doug's story …

Doug shared his experience of supporting his wife in higher care a few years ago. Doug talked about his sadness between tears. He believed she no longer recognised him or even realised he was there. He was down and despondent. He could no longer see any value in the visits and questioned whether there was even any point in visiting at all.

Doug spoke openly and from the heart. It was sad to hear the disconnect he felt from his wife whom he dutifully visited on a regular basis. We talked together about the role he could play and the new relationship that could be formed with his wife. It would look different to the one previously shared, but it would provide his wife with warmth and security, knowing someone cared about her and give him a sense of purpose. It was important to restore some sort of connection for them both. We explored the idea of a memory box with treasured mementos that he could bring when he visited her.

The box didn't need to be overly big and didn't need to contain a lot of items. They could be items his wife could safely hold or they could be items he could show her and reminisce about. They could be items that prompted his memory of stories they'd shared over a lifetime and ones he could recount out loud to her. Doug's face lit up; he was experiencing a sense of hope. He began listing off things he could use and include and why they were important to them both. The sadness in Doug's eyes transformed into joy within a matter of minutes and was truly humbling. He finally had a way forward; one he felt he could direct and control.

The Dementia Doula is best placed to create a space for individuals to come together and work out what they can provide to the person they're supporting. So many complaints and friction come from family members who feel unheard and disempowered, who lack the ability to say frankly what they want or need, how hurt they're feeling. A Dementia Doula can provide a safe opportunity for these discussions to take place in a no holds barred environment. They can support the venting of frustrations and perceived shortfalls in a therapeutic manner. Children are encouraged to be actively included in family discussions, when appropriate, and can offer valued insights. If we ever need an example of uncomplicated dementia care, just watch the innocent interactions of a child. They don't over think, and they don't overcompensate; they connect from the heart and follow wherever that takes them.

Thinking we're overthinking …

I once had an opportunity to do dementia training for a group of Year 7 students. They were about to visit an aged care home as part of a community service subject they were undertaking and would primarily be working with residents with dementia. I was there to provide some insight into dementia and some tips they could use for their interactions with residents. The session was well received by the students, and it was wonderful to see their interest in what was for many not only new subject material but also an experience they had not yet encountered firsthand.

I concluded the training with a discussion on the unpredictable nature of dementia and the expressions of emotions someone might show for reasons not always obvious or apparent to us at the time. I shared that they may be connecting with a resident who may shed tears or start to cry. I wanted to reassure the students they were unlikely to be at fault or have done something wrong. Their interactions may have reminded the person of someone from long ago or the person may feel overwhelmed with emotion in the moment.

I continued to emphasise that if this was to occur, they were not to blame. We discussed strategies for dealing with such a situation and I recommended they just let a nurse, or their teacher know what had happened. With that a young boy put his arm straight up in the air and said, 'But couldn't we just put our arm around them?'. It was in that moment I reflected on how complicated dementia care can become and not because of the disease itself. When we find ourselves in a caring role, we often feel desperate to try to find what's gone wrong, search for answers and try to fix things. This was such an innocent response but one with an amazing depth. It was one that went back to the concept of kindness, not overthinking a situation, but responding from the heart.

As mentioned several times throughout this book, when we refer to being the voice for those without, it isn't just the person with dementia, it's their unheard families who try to navigate the unknown in the only way they know how. They turn up every day, every week, every fortnight, every month and sometimes every year hoping that today things might make a bit more sense. The role of the Dementia Doula is to make today the day where everything comes together, and to replicate it tomorrow, along with the next day and the next. A Dementia Doula helps families look after themselves, to be kind to themselves, to not feel guilty when a day off is due, to see that being there 24/7 doesn't define connection or whether they care. To show that what's important is the connection they feel to the person or the version they once knew. Families don't give up caring, they give up because of the frustration that they can't fix, because they can't physically, mentally, or emotionally cope any longer, or because their hearts are broken, and they can no longer bear the pain.

Importance of everyone on the same page

By bringing everyone together, we're collectively more able to pave the way forward, to better focus on capturing the individual experiences of family members and staff and identify perceived limitations with current palliative care provision. Together it's easier to identify unknown variables and common themes that may emerge and require consideration when creating a solid foundation for everyone to start from. Everyone involved then becomes better placed to explore and identify the roadblocks they face.

Preparing in a timely way for death can be done with a level of certainty, with clear directives in place for when things happen or begin to unfold, or symptoms need managing. Families are often told how lucky they are when their family member has moved into supported care. There's a perception they're now free to do as they want, free from the perceived burden of caring. But needing to care doesn't just disappear for families. They don't resign from the caring role. It's a position they take on for life and nothing changes that, not even a family member relocating to a new environment. Family members continue to be an underutilised resource. However, including and acknowledging them as a vital part of our dynamic palliative care team is essential for moving forward into the future as a united front.

Equipping families with the language to converse with medical professionals and staff in a way that brings meaning and understanding will assist families in logically coming to their own conclusions based on the person's medical history and their life experiences. Clearly defined roles leave no question about what part they'll play, for families will no longer need representing because Dementia Doulas ensure they can do it for themselves. And if there's a wobbly moment, a Dementia Doula is there to help them stand straight again. A Dementia Doula doesn't make the decisions and doesn't encourage a certain path to be taken; the Dementia Doula simply clears the debris from the path so thinking and direction become a bit easier to navigate.

Team approach

When we look at a situation from a different perspective, what seemed to be a problem or issue, may be a simple misunderstanding. In dementia care there is a risk of looking for complex answers and solutions to something which at face value appears to be a complex issue. Coming together on a united front can bring perspective from many different angles. By implementing a team approach, there's a shared problem-solving ability with answers that may have been obvious all along. When a resident is perceived as 'the problem', taking a step back may reveal that was never actually the case.

Compassionate care means that a Dementia Doula needs to stay within a scope of practice but doesn't need to stick to a script, for when that happens, connection is so easily severed, and needs remain unmet. Dementia Doulas are flexible in thinking and can pivot with a moment's notice. Think about a well-meaning friend in your home, helping you in some way, maybe putting away some shopping. They're someone you've known for years and they're now in your environment helping you. Think for a moment how you'd feel looking at their face but not recognising them. They tell you that you do know them; they want you to remember, but you can't. Would it be wise for the friend to just continue going through your cupboards or should they adapt their approach and find a place of connection?

Without a team approach in place the consequences will be:

Someone with dementia will become a perceived 'problem' when support and nurturing is lacking, when needs aren't met, when the person isn't recognised for who they are at the core, for what they have to give or where they fit into the world.

Family members will become a perceived 'problem' when support and nurturing is lacking, when needs aren't met, when the person isn't recognised for who they are at the core, for what they have to give or where they fit into the world.

Staff will become a perceived 'problem' when support and nurturing is lacking, when needs aren't met, when the person isn't recognised for who they are at the core, for what they have to give or where they fit into the world.

This is an area where Dementia Doulas can make such a difference and generate a real sense of connection for families, not just with their family member with dementia, but with those supporting their care. They can help the support network look beyond what is happening to the physical aspects of a person and to look deeper and listen to the hidden messages within, to better explore the emotional needs of the person and see where there are new opportunities for connection. They provide a service that encompasses not only the person but those surrounding them.

As Dementia Doulas, we bring back hope and provide an opportunity to be heard, to be understood. It's about finding solace and a way to make peace with a life lived and the uncertainty of a complex future. It's hope that allows for better understanding of a situation brought about by an emptiness and fear, hurtful things that may be said or the pain left by a vacant stare. But there is hope for that which was no longer thought possible - being able to leave this world with nothing unresolved and the knowledge that those left behind will be ok. Bringing back hope isn't focussed on better future outcomes or better times ahead but instead on a new way of connecting that had seemed all but lost.

When supporting someone with dementia and attempting to problem solve an issue or understand a behaviour they may be exhibiting, it isn't always necessary to try to change the person themselves. The importance is often in changing the circumstances surrounding them. By working as a team, I've often discovered staff collectively hold the elusive key we're searching for, a key they unknowingly possess missing its true value and potential.

Anna's story ...

Anna was a Hungarian lady with advancing dementia who experienced distressing and agitated behaviours for which no one could determine the origins. It had been reported that Anna was agitated, aggressive, hoarding, refusing to eat, and stealing. These were the terms shared with me and were thought to be part of her dementia. With staff in a group session, we spent time exploring life with dementia to try to see life from Anna's perspective. We thought about how Anna was trying to purposefully connect with the environment surrounding her. It was evident we needed to explore who Anna was at her core.

Together with staff, we began putting together the jigsaw of her life. It appeared that staff all seemed to know individual pieces about Anna, but conflicting versions of her life quickly began to emerge. Some staff knew more about Anna than others. What we attempted to do was bring all the individual pieces together so we could step back and look at a bigger and more complete picture.

When staff got the idea of what we were trying to do, they started connecting her behaviours and responses to the life she'd shared with her husband and children. But something was still missing. We explored her life as a mother and grandmother and her constantly asking about her children. Loud sounds would startle and frighten her, and staff were fixated on the issues they had with her hoarding. The 'stealing' and 'hiding' of food in her wardrobe was something they weren't sure how to 'fix'. She carried a plastic shopping bag around, but this had been taken from her as it wasn't deemed appropriate.

The information contributed by staff, in their individual pieces, was quite interesting but nothing was giving away any clues as to why Anna was responding the way she did and the theories behind her behaviours weren't quite fitting. I encouraged staff to think deeper and more broadly, to give me something they knew about Anna but perhaps thought not relevant or significant. I wanted ANYTHING.

It was then we struck gold. A staff member raised her hand and said she thought Anna had grown up somewhere in Eastern Europe during the war. She said she knew nothing more than that. What this did though was to prompt another staff member to add further to Anna's story and provide the key we'd been searching for. From that moment, everything changed. This staff member shared that she knew Anna had lived in Eastern Europe during World War II. She and her younger siblings had become orphaned during the war and as a young teenager she became the primary carer not only for herself but also her two younger sisters. They had been homeless and lived on the streets.

This new insight sent chills through everyone and left us all feeling teary as the true picture of Anna's world started to unfold. We took a moment to process what we'd just heard and the implications. Staff began connecting the dots and realised the children Anna was searching for were likely her younger siblings and not her adult children. Her need to hoard food made more sense along with her fear of sudden and loud noises. They realised Anna was spending every moment of every day in survival mode, trying to stay safe and to provide for her siblings.

It was through this opportunity to bring Anna to life in a way staff could connect with that brought everyone on the same page and together they began brainstorming how they could better support her. One staff member even suggested giving her back her plastic shopping bag so she could collect things throughout the day. They even thought of ways to assist her with her hoarding and if it was food, they'd simply remove it from her wardrobe when she was sleeping.

Staff had unknowingly held vital pieces of the puzzle but needed the opportunity and a forum through which to bring the jigsaw of Anna's life together. Staff started to see how difficult and traumatic daily life in the care home had become and was continuing to be for Anna. But the difference now was that they knew they could be a part of the solution.

A Dementia Doula is best placed to step forward and start those conversations, ensuring everyone involved understands and knows the person's story from the very start. Take Anna's story. A Dementia Doula would continue to bring Anna's story to life in a way that staff and her family could better connect with. They would continue connecting them to it when Anna needed it most so that they are able to prepare Anna indirectly for what is to come through briefing and preparing those who surround her on a day-to-day basis.

Families will never truly know or understand the life of their loved one, as close as they may be. Think of your relationship with your own children, partners, siblings, parents. Think about how much they know of your life, of your history, what your earlier years of life looked like and from whose perspective. Who brings that important information to the forefront when it's needed, when the time is right? It's here a Dementia Doula is well placed to assist, playing an investigative role, being a detective, piecing together the past of someone's life as it's known in parts by different individuals. They can establish what life looked like for them at any given time, even if it starts with a generalised framework, helping staff and families understand what the person sees and perceives around them.

Mentoring & role models

Mentoring and being a role model is to be the best version of you, fulfilling a role it's hoped others will want to emulate. It's not about creating clones. It's about taking qualities of a job and putting one's own personal spin on them. It's to influence and inspire others, hoping they might consider a different way forward, but to do so personalising those attributes to who they are and inject their own personality into the mix, to develop but to continue functioning as themselves, being their own true self and being genuine in how they come across.

A Dementia Doula can assist with ongoing professional practice development of staff providing a dementia context, facilitating valuable discussions and resources for enhancing their practices. Let me share my own stories of inspiration from early in my own career as I explored who I wanted to be as a nurse. It was the practice of two colleagues at different stages that influenced my practice in a way they'll never truly appreciate and all because they were just being themselves.

Through my eyes …

I first worked with Sam in a care home as I went through my nursing training. Sam was a care assistant and a few years younger than me and working with her was something I looked forward to. She had an ability to make work fun. She had a beautiful smile and a natural connection with residents. She was genuine and heartfelt. I enjoyed seeing faces literally light up when she entered the rooms of residents. She was playful when appropriate and toned it down when required. To me, every resident saw her as a proxy granddaughter and that's just the way they responded and connected with her. I knew I wanted to build this type of connection with patients moving forward in my career. I couldn't pull it off like Sam did, but I knew I could create the 'me' version. I wanted to tap into the same essence that Sam had. She never hid behind a title, instead she brought her true self to the experience of others, and they trusted her as I saw them trust no other.

After graduating from university, I found myself working with Merridy on a fast-paced surgical ward where there wasn't time for the 'niceties' Sam had taught me. This was a lesson in process and getting things done in a timely manner. There was no time to provide the care I so desperately wanted to. I'd watch Merridy, an enrolled nurse who bought calmness and serenity to otherwise chaotic situations. She would connect quickly and genuinely with patients and their families, and she helped me realise those qualities I'd been consciously bringing to the fore could be adapted to any situation. Without compromising efficiency, Merridy maintained a warmth, a kindness and calmness that not only reassured her patients they would be alright but also that she was by their side. She brought a comfort to her patients and their family members that was genuinely seen in their faces which would light up when she entered the room. I, too, wanted to emulate these qualities not only as a nurse but also in my Paramedic role. It was Merridy who showed me I could still leave patients feeling reassured and comforted even in a fast paced, emergency situation.

I believed I was already the best version of me, but after meeting and observing these two amazing women, two of my role models, so early on in my career, I knew I had the ability to be more. Both women were instrumental in the development of who I wanted to be and how I wanted to connect with others. They both consistently demonstrated a professionalism many others struggle with today.

They incorporated and mixed in perfect amounts of kindness and connection. They were authentic, empathetic and had a fitting sense of humour. They were personable, friendly, and went the extra mile doing things a person needed without even being asked. They got to know the person. They got to know their families and they made it a priority to know what was important to them all. They could be in the moment with someone, where time appeared to slow down around them.

They taught me the importance of not losing sight of what I brought to the table, that I didn't have to create a professional persona to gain trust and credibility. I just needed to be me, the me that others could easily connect with, the me that others knew they could trust. The best part was they made me want to be the best version of myself. I wanted to emulate them but still genuinely be the 'me' version. Patients were still people with basic human needs, who needed to be respected, heard, and cared about and treated in a dignified way. They taught me that regardless of time pressures and deadlines.

I have no doubt these two women had no idea of the impact they were having on me and why would they? After all, they were just being themselves, and that's why it's so important to be the type of person that will inspire others to find their gifts, to be conscious of how they'll act and respond. If we rush or appear rushed then all those around us will follow suit, chaos will undoubtedly ensue, and the person gets lost in the crowd. Just keep in mind with whatever you do, you'll never know who's watching.

The Dementia Doula, as a mentor, taps into that special something within many that's needed to bring out the added extras, to help others to navigate and negotiate a rudderless system, being persuasive when required and showing professionalism. The strength is in going it alone, fuelled by the coming together of other likeminded individuals, discovering what's inside.

Getting staff on board

If we want to get staff on board, we need to speak their language, to understand and acknowledge the everyday challenges and limitations they face and be conscious that anything we do needs to clearly state what's in it for them. Staff won't buy into anything they think will make their job more complicated or be time consuming. They won't enjoy being made to feel that others want to tell them how they can do their job better. The job of a Dementia Doula is to support and encourage staff and ultimately make their life easier, to walk alongside them providing insight and context for the everyday situations they face. The intent is not to burden them with greater expectations or responsibilities, but to provide a way to support them better, in turn, lightening their load. Dementia Doulas keep it real with families and need to do the same with staff. Dementia Doulas aren't out to impress but to just keep showing up when needed and be in the background when they're not.

By incorporating more relationship-centred practices into care home settings ensures better service delivery while promoting dignity and compassion. When we bring a practical and relationship-centred focus to care, we can start to influence positive change. Together we can tackle the issues associated with someone entering higher care, bringing their expectations of care to life, creating a better understanding for those involved in facilitating the process.

It is unreasonable to expect new residents to just 'settle in', to pick up, adopt and conform to a new set of rules they're expected to live by, the behaviour expected of them within the new environment, and all this with compromised cognition and no rule book to follow. It's such a disconnect and I've often asked staff how their 'transitioning into care' program works, knowing I'm likely to receive a blank or confused look. I ask what their organisational policy is for new residents or respite clients, what they do to ensure there's a smooth transition into the care environment. Historically I've been met with, 'We don't have one'. How is that fair to the person with dementia, their families or even to staff? The Dementia Doula is well placed to support this time of transition for all and at the very least have everyone on the same page.

Sometimes the level of expectation is too high for someone living with dementia to easily adapt to a new environment. Add to this the trauma and unsettledness associated with any type of relocation along with the lack of a consistent transitioning process. Imagine turning up day one to a new job, with new surroundings to navigate, new faces to remember, feeling disoriented and unable to initiate the simplest of tasks - not even being sure where the bathroom is or where to get a cup of tea and looking forward to going home because you're feeling so overwhelmed.

Imagine starting that new job without any orientation program, where you were just expected to blend in and do the 'right thing', to know where you're meant to be and what you're meant to be doing. You would surely think this unreasonable and be expecting some support in learning what the new job was about along with the associated systems, to be briefed on the processes informing the expectations of the role.

While such an in depth and formalised process isn't going to be suitable for someone living with dementia entering care, they still deserve something, a process to meet their needs in that moment, and for the moments that follow, one where their families are included. This is an everchanging environment that will continue to be everchanging so getting everyone on the same page as soon as possible will set the tone of a better experience for all.

Question for reflection …

As a role model, when others look at you would they be inspired by what they see?

The gift …

When focussing on the person as an individual it assists in keeping us accountable. It's knowing there's someone out there depending on us and that's extremely motivating.

I know what I can do now, I'll put together his story before he goes into care and then staff will understand him better.

• Family member •

9 • Support as the end draws near

'It is reported that, given the right support, most people would prefer to die at home, yet a very small minority of people with dementia do so.'

-   Mogan et. al., 2018, p.1042

Supporting families and someone with dementia at the end of their life is such a humbling experience for a Dementia Doula; to be part of intimate, precious and sacred conversations when the time comes. A Dementia Doula is prepared for these difficult conversations and does so in a nurturing and sensitive way. Often by avoiding these conversations, families are left to continue connecting the dots and making it up as they go along. By opening these doors for families, a Dementia Doula better prepares them for the uncertainties of dementia, and the challenges they're likely to face.

Families who are better prepared for what's to come are more united and feel less alone. Dementia Doulas have their own narrative that will serve them well to connect with the aged care industry. Conversations carry weight for all involved and it's important to be clear and use carefully chosen words. The following story is an example of conversations that were well-intentioned but resulted in a disconnection for those involved.

Glady's story …

I was on a nightshift at a care home where Gladys, a long-term resident, still lay awake at 1am in the morning. She was unsettled but unable to articulate or pinpoint why. While Gladys was experiencing early dementia, it was mobility issues that saw her requiring higher care. It had become apparent over the previous few weeks that Gladys was nearing the end of her life. I chose to sit with Gladys during my shift break. We sat in quietness with only her bedside lamp on and I asked what she had on her mind. She replied, 'Why won't God take me? Why aren't I good enough?'.

Gladys wasn't actively practicing a faith, but this was a time, in the quiet and stillness of the night where she lay thinking of where her place was in the world. She was suffering physically, often struggling to find a comfortable position and she was sad that this was how her life was ending. I wasn't sure what to say but continued to chat with Gladys. I wanted to understand what was going on for her. Gladys continued talking with sadness about not being worthy and being made to suffer. I could see there was more she wanted to say so I asked her directly whether there was anything holding her back from dying, and she replied, 'My sister-in-law visited a few days ago and I told her I wanted to die, that I was ready', and her reply was, 'No, you'll be fine, you're not going anywhere, we still need you here'.

There it was, a simple statement that had impacted Gladys in ways I'm sure weren't intended. She lacked permission to 'go', and it seemed she was hanging on for her family. We chatted further and I felt humbled to be able to share in that time with Gladys, to help her find a sense of peace about dying, that others would be okay and would understand she had to go. Most importantly, she wouldn't be letting anyone down. A couple of days later Gladys died, and I felt a sense of relief that her wish for peace had been granted.

While Glady's experience is not common for someone with dementia, to be able to share their thoughts and feelings in the latter stage, the principles remain the same - what is said and words that are used, and more importantly how they are said and how they are processed by the person until the end. A Dementia Doula is in the privileged position to be able to guide families at this emotional time and bring about a plan for how this time will unfold. The earlier this is captured, the better. Even if it's captured later, a Dementia Doula can still guide this conversation and invite families to contribute in ways they feel most comfortable.

The Dementia Doula will play a pivotal role in how prepared families feel in being beside their loved one as they're dying or during the lead up to death. The ultimate goal is to support the person with dementia in experiencing a peaceful death surrounded by those closest to them with four key areas of care being addressed. These include physical comfort, mental and emotional needs, spiritual needs, and practical tasks. Of course, the family of the dying person needs support as well, especially with practical tasks and emotional distress. Preparing families is about bringing them together and guiding them through the creation of an end-stage setting that's conducive to a place of calmness and peace, having conversations with families if they haven't happened already about what's to come, along with what they may face and experience.

The importance of a Dementia Doula helping families to prepare for this time can't be stressed enough. When more difficult conversations may have been had earlier, this becomes a time where families can be encouraged to relax, rest and just be in the moment, to prepare for what's to come. These previous conversations now become essential as they can mean the difference between someone with dementia dying in the comfort of their own surroundings or result in them being sent to hospital. When staff are supported by knowing where to access tailored Advance Care Directives, family then have time to put measures in place for how the end-of-life stage will play out. Dementia Doulas assist families in understanding that dying is not a clinical event but a normal part of life. This is highlighted in the following story about Peter.

Peter's story …

I was presenting a family session within a high care setting. All had gone smoothly with good interaction from the group. As the session concluded, Peter came to speak to me on his own. He shared how difficult it had been watching his mother continue to deteriorate and he felt he lacked understanding of what was going on for her. In a poignant moment for me Peter said, 'This was all well and good and I learnt heaps tonight, but this was more like what I needed to know when Mum first came into care. What I need from someone like you now is to know where we're heading with all this. What's coming? Because I've got no idea. I want to know what we're supposed to be doing.'

I smiled at Peter and nodded in agreement and told him I couldn't have agreed with him more. This is where the system has let families down. A lot of information is provided in the earlier stages thinking families will sift through what's relevant at that point in time and come back to it when it's needed at some stage in the future. But it's not usually tailored to the experience of the individual on a given day.

The need for better communication at end-of-life

There will be many occasions where there hasn't been an opportunity for earlier discussions to have taken place within families or with the person with dementia themselves. Conversations with families and a Dementia Doula must be factored in regardless of the time frame to prepare them for what's to come, even if death is imminent. Relationship and trust building becomes paramount and will likely to be done with an element of haste. A Dementia Doula will still need to create the opportunity for end-of-life discussions and do it in a sensitive and unambiguous way.

The Dementia Doula role supports existing research suggesting more in-depth conversations are required for families to fully understand, and be best placed for navigating, the final stages of dementia. While research strongly suggests health professionals should be incorporating these conversations into their existing practice, the reality is they often lack capacity or time to do so. These are conversations requiring a sensitive approach with honest dialogue and should ideally not be rushed.

As a Dementia Doula we are best placed to have these conversations in a way that conveys empathy, compassion, honesty, and a sense of hope; to discuss concerns and sensitive issues on a regular basis with family members encouraging them to ask questions and relay their wishes. As part of their ongoing role, and particularly if they are part of a care home staffing model, a Dementia Doula can then check in with family members to ensure continuing understanding of the information provided and find where it sits for them at any given time. When death is imminent families are then better prepared for what's to come and how it's likely to play out. To ensure respect and dignity of family members it is vital to acknowledge that they will all differ in the amount of information they wish to be privy to and the role they're wanting to play.

An uncomfortable silence

Death is a difficult topic to discuss. However, the lack of discussion sees everyone making it up as they go along or when facing it head on when the time ultimately comes. Anticipated fears can make this significant time in our lives differ from all the others. Think about a party you're hosting. Do you let a few people informally know it's on and hope someone turns up? Do you not bother to sort out catering because it might get too complicated with all the dietary requirements, and you don't want to risk offending someone? What do you do then when a bunch of random people turn up at your door because you didn't specify a date or time? With a baby on the way, is it worth sorting out how the process will unfold? Would a doctor be involved, or would we just wing that too?

Typically speaking, we don't make up the details in significant life events as they're unfolding. We plan and revise the plan, making sure everyone who is involved is on the same page. We ensure people know what role they'll play and how they'll go about it. Why then do we commonly leave the details of death and dying to chance? If we keep the blinkers on, do we secretly hope we might just stop it from happening?

The Dementia Doula needs to feel comfortable about having conversations around death and dying with their clients. We can only do this successfully and genuinely if we're first prepared to have those conversations with ourselves and know where this sits for us. If I use me as a starting point and feel comfortable with the dialogue, then I'm less inclined to sound all doom and gloom or uncomfortable when I initiate the conversation with others. This is a milestone of life that shouldn't be regarded or discussed any differently to any other we go through. As you read through my reflections, I invite you to think about your own. Jot down some notes if you want to. Don't skip to the next chapter. I promise you; this is a conversation worth having.

Sharing my thoughts …

I don't mind a bit of control in my life at any time, so why would dying be any different? A good death for me would be in having as much control as possible over the final stage of my life. But for others it can mean something totally different and that's why conversations must happen much earlier to ensure these thoughts are captured. I would hope for opportunities in directing and personalising my care or if that's not the scenario, that when my time came it was quick and without suffering or pain.

Key elements for me would be having choice, options, empowerment, and comfort. Personalised care would assist me in feeling in control of how things progressed and ensure I didn't become just a number. I'd want to be surrounded by a team of professionals that understood my wishes and what was important to me. I've nursed many patients with debilitating conditions who would quietly confide they wish they'd died because of the event that took their quality of life away.

A good death for me would be about choice about how that stage would look and flow, to have input into every aspect of care and the circumstances surrounding it, to be able to say what I want and when I want it, knowing there is no 'one size fits all' approach or treatment regime for end-of-life care. Choice for me would also include deciding for myself when enough was enough and explore ALL other options. My palliative care team would ultimately include an End-of-Life-Doula or a Dementia Doula if relevant. I would ensure my team were aware they played a strong advocacy role also.

I would have a list of things that are important to me, my 'non negotiables', and things I may be more flexible about. I wouldn't want any of my wishes to be thought of as 'nice to have' or come second to clinical interventions, unless of course it's pain relief. I would have listed medications and treatments I may want or need and any medications that haven't sat well with me in the past. I would want the right to decline treatment, medications or life sustaining care or have a nominated person advocate on my behalf. I want those responsible for my care to respect my Advance Care Directives and ensure my wishes are acted upon. I'd not want to prolong unnecessary suffering, not only for myself but for my loved ones too.

It would be important to me that I'm treated as a person and not the disease or condition I may appear to have become. I've witnessed many patients and residents in the past referred to as the 'stroke in room 3' or 'the dementia in room 10'. It may sometimes be the actual words used but on other occasions it's been the tone of voice or clinical nature of words used that can still impact on personhood and a sense of normality. It can be difficult at times for those in a caring position to see past the hospital gown or flannelette pyjamas.

My ultimate wish is for comfort - surrounded by family and friends knowing quietness is important to me, as are places that bring me peace and help me to mentally detach from the craziness of a fast-paced world: places that bring me feelings of connection and emotional comfort and maintain my daily rituals and routines including loose leaf English Breakfast tea with a generous dash of milk. Who would know that if I didn't capture it in some way?

For me, as you can see, a good death is not just one thing. It's a culmination of key elements such as options available to me, choices I have, how empowered I feel, and the need for those things that bring me comfort. Being empowered in decision making or having an ability to delegate that responsibility all come together and would give me a sense of control. This control is over my ultimate destiny, how I'd want to leave this world.

So why would any of this be different for someone living with dementia? It's not. It highlights the need to encourage this type of conversation happening sooner rather than later. And when I say encourage, I don't mean handing over a bunch of brochures and saying, 'You need to fill these out'. I mean taking someone through the process in a way that they can better connect with, one that meets them where they're at today and points them in the direction for what they're likely to experience or face next.

If it's too difficult for a family to consider speaking on behalf of their family member, then perhaps, for clarity, invite them to reflect inwardly and think about what's important to them. This is a topic where a sensitive manner is essential for starting conversations that may not be a normal part of a family's everyday dialogue. Regardless, it's an important conversation to have because when the time comes a Dementia Doula wants to feel assured that families know there will ultimately be no rules. Instead, it will be a time for families to take a breath and navigate through instinctively, not waiting for permission to do something, or hold back because they feel it's the right thing to do.

Families need to feel encouraged to follow what feels comfortable and right for them. We need to create opportunities for them to be a part of something it's hoped will bring comfort and a sense of peace as they work towards their own sense of closure, to assist them to take the opportunity to tell the person with dementia they are loved one last time, always assuming the person can still hear them until the end.

Providing comfort and care for someone during their end-of-life stage can be physically and emotionally exhausting. A Dementia Doula will encourage families to ask for help when it's needed or accept help when it's offered, and not to hesitate in suggesting specific tasks to someone offering any form of assistance. Friends and family are often eager to support those in a frontline position but often don't know what that could look like. A Dementia Doula can provide a list of tasks or errands they may choose from which could include things like:

- Being there to talk to over a coffee
- Small daily jobs around the house
- Picking up mail
- Doing some laundry
- Taking family members out for an hour or two break
- Offering to sit with the person with dementia while family attend to other things
- Coordinating those offering assistance
- Taking the dog for a walk and feeding pets
- Doing some shopping
- Looking after children
- Preparing meals of homemade comfort food

As the end draws near

Preparing families for a bedside vigil will be easier to discuss as a type of process but the reality will be something far more fluid in nature. By providing a checklist type format it can help families grasp where they may want to position themselves during this time and how they'd like to be involved. It allows opportunity for conversations to happen at a time not highly emotive or stressful.

The following are suggestions only and may be of use to a Dementia Doula in preparing their clients or initiating the conversation. They may be adapted for individual circumstances and only intended as a starting point. Remind families to always remember to check with staff to ensure any interventions are appropriate and safe.

1. Pain management: Ultimately there's a need for the person to not physically suffer in any way. Families may be best placed to observe when the person doesn't appear comfortable or is in pain. If families are made aware of some of the signs possibly indicating pain, medications can be administered earlier rather than later, minimising suffering and ensuring as much comfort as possible. If the person is shifting around the bed or restless, if they scrunch up their face into a grimace with or without touch, or their limbs contract in a muscle spasm, then families should feel comfortable in notifying staff that pain management is required.

2. Mouth hygiene: During the final stages of dying, mouth breathing is likely. The person's mouth will dry out quickly and be uncomfortable. In consultation with staff, families may want to be involved in the swabbing of the person's mouth with swabs provided by staff to ensure the mouth is kept moist. A suitable lip balm may also be applied.

3. Cleaning the person during the vigil: Family may feel comfortable gently washing the persons face, neck, arms, hands, feet, and legs with a lukewarm damp cloth. A light, non-

fragranced moisturiser could then gently be massaged into the person's face, hands, arms, legs, and feet. It must be emphasised that this activity may not be suitable for everyone because of sensory changes experienced by the person due to dementia, so taking the lead from the person and how they respond to the sensation is vital. If any discomfort is noted, cleaning and massage should be ceased all together. Awareness should also be drawn to delicate skin areas where dabbing of the skin rather than rubbing would be recommended to avoid skin tears.

4. Peaceful environment: Keeping the room quiet and lowering the lighting if possible, using lamps or battery-operated candles, ensures a calmness and peacefulness for the person. Encourage those who enter the person's space to speak softly with no loud noises, no harsh lights, and an awareness of language being used. It's important for those around the person to speak *to* them and not *about* them in their presence. Limit the number of people present at any one time.

5. Time out: The dying person will not require family to be by their side constantly and it's important for them to have quiet time. Families will need their own rest to sustain them for the unknown number of hours or days ahead. Encourage families to go for regular walks outside, to get fresh air, go home for a period, go out for a meal, or talk with others outside of the room.

6. Fresh air: There may be some cultural considerations for opening a window if possible and these are conversations to have with families. Keeping the air in the room as fresh as possible could be considered if practical to do so. Overly fragrant flowers can be overwhelming and should be discouraged altogether. A small fan may be considered to help with air movement and ambient temperature control.

7. Observing religious or spiritual needs: Religious and/or spiritual rites are important for many people as part of their dying process. Earlier discussions with family members should establish if the person would want a visit from a religious or spiritual advisor and when to ensure this is enacted for them.

8. Talk to the person: Encourage families to talk to the dying person or read to them. There will likely be an awareness for the person that others are present. Prompt the sharing of special memories or experiences shared together. Encourage families to speak from the heart, from a place of compassion, but explain it's not helpful to bring up hurt or past wrongs. The person with dementia is unlikely to have context for such conversations and may become distressed.

9. Music: Music tailored to the person or relaxation may be appropriate and played only intermittently. When playing music, ensure it is done so quietly and discourage others from talking at the same time. Advise families to be aware of speaker placement and to not put them too close to the person's head/ears. Music must be used with caution as the person requires a quiet and tranquil space.

10. Keeping a journal: If family are taking it in turns to be with the person or others will be visiting at different times, it may be useful to keep a journal on hand. Those visiting will then have the opportunity to write down that they visited, at what time and on which day. They may document what they did with or for the person and whether there was any response, positive or negative. This will give the next person something to build on and give an indication as to whether they've already had a lot of visitors on a given day.

Signs that someone is dying

Each death will be different, but as the person nears end of life there are likely to be common signs. Physical changes don't occur in any specific order and are an indication the body's systems are shutting down. These are likely to include:

- sleeping more
- eating and drinking less
- breathing changes, which can sound rattly, irregular and laboured
- hallucinations and sleep disturbances
- restless moving, twitching, groaning
- cool skin, especially the hands and feet
- dry mouth and dry or cracked lips
- noticeable discolouration of skin

Witnessing these changes can be distressing for families, so speaking with them earlier and preparing them for what they are likely to see will assist them with processing how comfortable they feel being involved. Reassure families that these symptoms will and can be adequately managed by staff.

When the person has died

A Dementia Doula can let families know that it's okay to take time to sit with the person's body once they've died as part of the process of letting them go. There's no hurry, and families can stay until they're ready to say their final goodbyes.

Some may want to wait until other family members or friends have attended and had an opportunity to also say goodbye. Some families may feel comfortable with washing the body in preparation for ongoing funeral arrangements, others will not.

Reassure them there is no right or wrong in this decision. If they wish to, they can be guided by staff if available.

Remembering the person

Due to the drawn-out nature of dying for someone living with dementia, families may struggle with the moment of death, given they've been losing the person often over many years. Encourage families to mark the moment and time by doing something special to acknowledge and honour their life. This may assist family members in transitioning into the bereavement phase and assist them with their loss.

- Frame a photo, cherished note or other memento
- Cook their favourite meal or cake
- Plant a special tree or flower
- Light a candle
- Organise to have a memorial plaque put in a favourite spot
- Make a contribution to their preferred charity or community group
- Create an online memorial page with photos and stories
- Visit a favourite venue and bring along a special memento

Brian's story …

Visiting a favourite venue following the death of a loved one reminds me of a story shared by Brian's family from chapter 1. Following his death, Brian's family went for dinner at his favourite restaurant and took along his treasured hat, a hat he was known to wear daily. The hat took pride of place, on its own seat at the table, leaving family feeling as though he'd joined them for a final meal together.

As the end draws nearer, the Dementia Doula can work alongside families and staff creating an environment conducive to spreading a sense of calm and peace for everyone involved and one for setting the scene of what's to come. With conversations already had, and plans well documented, there should be no need for panic or last-minute hospital admissions (unless there's other medical considerations). Panic often comes from lack of a role or sense of purpose, but that's what the Dementia Doula prepares everyone for, ensuring no one goes it alone.

Question for reflection …

How does someone living with dementia find peace and resolution particularly in the later stages?

The gift …

For someone with advanced dementia, it's never over until it's over. Make today count, make the moments matter.

'A Dementia Doula doesn't ask if something can be done but instead why can't it be?'

• Dementia Doula •

10 • A new path awaits

'… findings would support development of an intervention to help people with dementia and their families and carers have facilitated discussions about these issues of future place of care earlier in the illness …'

- Lord et. al., 2016, p.7

We, as Dementia Doulas, are in the perfect position to make the necessary changes today that will influence what dementia care looks like tomorrow, and into the future. If we don't influence change as we have the capacity to do, then the future of dementia care will continue to look strikingly similar to what it does to today. The certainty is that this is a sector unlikely to receive any huge increases to funding or staffing levels any time soon. Given the increase in predicted numbers of those living with dementia in Australia climbing from 470,000 today to 1.1 million by 2051 (Dementia Australia, 2022), we need to realise how things look now could actually be as good as they're likely to get.

It doesn't need to be this way. Dementia Doulas can ensure this isn't the way the future unfolds. We can bring light to an ever-dark path. Care can and must be tailored to the individual and their support networks. If we are led by the words and actions received from someone living with dementia, then we'll know what needs to be done. Our responses and reactions are pivotal to how everyday exchanges will pan out, whether everyone gets frustrated and gives up or keeps on trying to find a different and better way to connect. There isn't a one size fits all approach due to how dementia impacts individuals. Therein lies the problem. We're attempting to communicate with another human living with various complexities and challenges. What we can ensure is at every turning point, there's a Dementia Doula waiting.

Walking the united path of change

Dementia Doulas are raising current industry standards by creating a valued and respected role that truly advocates for people with dementia, their families and care staff. They take words and put them into action in a unique way. Dementia Doulas assist in planning and creating a roadmap for the person living with dementia, and in doing so, it's hoped the path will be less daunting or overwhelming for all involved. The plan may need some adapting along the way, but knowing that the journey is shared, that potholes will be navigated together, will assist in future decision-making being smoother and easier.

This compassionate type of caring a Dementia Doula offers is shaping a new version of dementia care. There are so many individuals in the Dementia Doula space trying new things, following their instincts, and coming up with amazing concepts to support dementia care. They're more than just fun activities, they're about a quality of life for those living with advancing dementia and their families. It's about no longer waiting for someone higher up the food chain to sort things out. It's about asking ourselves, 'What's within my sphere of influence? What do I have to give that will make a difference?' Even the shortest of conversations can have an impact on others, helping them to see things from a different perspective. It doesn't have to be complicated or take a lot of planning.

A Dementia Doula ensures Compassionate care becomes part of everyday discussions and not left off any agenda. It has a front seat alongside clinical and personal care. It brings with it a new dialogue that can often be difficult to hear. It speaks in a way that can often bring tears but also a sense of clarity. Dementia Doulas ensure the dialogue leaves everyone knowing where they stand and why they've shown up. It's taking relationships back to the grass roots where expectation is clearly understood, where the principles of everyday life outside of dementia are employed inside the realm of dementia care.

Maintaining strength and resilience

The responsibilities of a Dementia Doula start with the Dementia Doula themselves. To ensure longevity within an industry that can be unrelenting and at times physically and emotionally draining, it's essential to be aware of one's own wellbeing. If wellbeing is not a consideration or made a priority, a Dementia Doula runs the risk of burn out with nothing more to give to others or themselves. By prioritising wellbeing as part of a personal daily practice, reserves can be built to draw upon when times become challenging. Being aware of one's individual needs sets a Dementia Doula up to create and maintain a good work/life balance.

Considerations should include:

- Staying current and industry relevant through ongoing learning opportunities
- Staying connected to a Dementia Doula community for support and direction
- Working within a defined role with clear professional and personal boundaries

Setting realistic expectations

A Dementia Doula can't be everything to everybody and nor should we try, because when we do, we stray outside the boundaries of our role and water down the very part of us that is unique and doing something pretty amazing in a very specialised space. We also place ourselves at risk of raising expectations and letting others down. Boundaries keep us safe and protect from physical and emotional overload. It's important that a Dementia Doula doesn't forget about themselves. In order to be who our clients need us to be, we must look after ourselves in a way that respects the complexity of the role we play in the lives of others.

A Dementia Doula works in a position that is giving on so many levels. It's a service that others need and take willingly. It would be remiss not to address the taxing nature of the role and ensure those entering or are currently within the field look after themselves. Prioritising our own wellbeing ensures we are available when our clients need us the most. As mentioned earlier, burnout is a very big issue within the aged care industry, and it's not well addressed within the sector. To avoid burnout, we need to recognise none of us have unlimited time or energy to give. Wellbeing recognises and identifies areas of our lives where we require additional support and develop strategies to maintain wellbeing. It's important not to be too hard on ourselves if there's a need for a break or to slow down in any way.

Great staff continue to leave the sector not because they don't care, but because they've got nothing more to give. We want to set Dementia Doulas up as best as we possibly can to ensure they build resilience and strength to draw on when times do become challenging, so they'll be there for today, tomorrow and the next day.

I just don't have time

'I just don't have time' are defining words for me. As soon as I think them or say them out loud, I'm hit instantly with a big reality check. When I say those words, it usually means I should make time for the thing I'm about to put on the back burner. Taking my dog for a walk in the local national park is one such time. I have a routine in place for when I go otherwise it wouldn't happen. I know myself too well. If I find I'm thinking I don't have time for a walk on that day, I can then identify I'm likely feeling out of sorts. It indicates that my thought processes are likely to be scattered and I'm likely feeling overwhelmed with the day ahead.

By making myself take the necessary steps to go for that walk, I'm able to clear the fog from my brain, to better compartmentalise aspects of my life that would otherwise stay sitting inside me in a jumbled heap. Thoughts that leave me stressing about what I need to do first, where might I start, begin to dissipate. Making time for a walk in our local national park is something that brings me a sense of clarity and peace and allows for that compartmentalising. It allows me to put things in their rightful place, the right storage container in my brain, so they're not only easier for me to see but also to access and address. The risk for me if I don't make time for my walk, is becoming overwhelmed, burnt out and unable to continue in a role I feel so passionate about.

Here's a quick and simple exercise to do. Turn to the front cover of this book and see if you could see yourself sitting on the Dementia Doula picnic rug. Take a few moments to picture yourself enjoying yummy food and a beverage, with not a care in the world. If your answer is, 'No, way!' or 'I wouldn't have time for a picnic', then maybe, you need to make time for a picnic! Think about how you would be feeling if you *were* sitting on that picnic rug and fully immersed in the moment. Would you perhaps feel calm and relaxed taking in the moment, enjoying the food, wine and company?

I think it's time we normalised self-care each day regardless of the wobbly bits in between. So, while you mightn't be a picnic kind of person, those feelings of being in the moment are 100% yours for the taking. I invite you once more to take another look at the cover, and if you aren't feeling like you can take time out for you, then change needs to start right now.

We want Dementia Doulas to be there for the long haul. This is a profession that speaks to and recognises a higher purpose. It creates a role that's exciting to turn up for every day. But if we don't prioritise ourselves, we run the risk of being exposed to, and consumed by, ongoing stressors, trying desperately to plug the holes draining our emotional energy and impacting on the relationships we work so hard to create. As Dementia Doulas we can be present over an extended period of time, depending on the wishes of a family. As such, we should regularly do a stock take on how we're feeling and identify areas likely to need attention.

Some common signs and symptoms to be aware of that may require support include:

- Feeling anxious, depressed, or irritable
- Feeling tired, run down with less energy
- Having difficulty with sleeping or exhaustion
- Overreacting to things usually considered minor
- Developing health issues (physical or mental)
- Having trouble concentrating
- Drinking, smoking, or eating more than usual
- Neglecting responsibilities or own needs
- Reduction in leisure activities
- Feeling helpless or hopeless

These are warning signs that it's time to take action and regain a sense of balance in our lives. If unattended to, when wellbeing is not considered a priority, Dementia Doulas place themselves at risk of compassion fatigue. Along with burnout, compassion fatigue is a type of stress resulting from regular exposure to working with grieving or traumatised individual/s rather than experiencing the grief or trauma first-hand.

The result is the person living in a state of physical and mental exhaustion with an inability to cope and function well with everyday tasks or within everyday environments. This can impact the high standard of care provided to clients as well as relationships with colleagues. If compassion fatigue is not addressed, there's the potential of more serious mental health conditions such as post-traumatic stress disorder (PTSD), anxiety or depression.

As Dementia Doulas we must be aware of the need to find ways to restore a sense of hope and joy, to give ourselves the chance to have a break and take time to recharge. As previously mentioned, if like me you hear yourself say you don't have time, it's likely a big red flag that you need to make time for you.

Some simple concepts to incorporate into the working day for ongoing self-care might include:

1. Asking for help – If you don't already have one, create a support network for yourself and your family if needed during peak times. Don't wait for others to guess how you're feeling or what you need. You don't have to do it all on your own. That's what we tell our clients, so we need to practise this in order to be authentic.

2. Spending time with friends - When we're busy and overworked or feeling stressed, often spending time with supportive friends isn't always a priority. But it can make all the difference. Maintaining friendships and social connections is essential for wellbeing and minimises the risk of feeling like you're going it alone. Even a phone call if it's too difficult to catch up in person can help.

3. Taking breaks each day - While caring can sometimes mean being on call 24/7, it's important that you allow yourself to take breaks every day and not feel guilty for taking days off from time to time. There is only so much you can do and sacrificing your own health and well-being doesn't help anyone. A break could be enjoying a coffee or meal, reading your favourite book, taking a walk, spending time with friends, or practising mindfulness.

4. Make time for hobbies – Hobbies provide an opportunity to slow down and reconnect with something else that's enjoyable to you. Hobbies can assist with retaining a sense of self and promote feelings of well-being and should always be on the priority list.

Jan's story ...

I'd worked with Jan over many years and could see the passion she felt working with families and those living with dementia. Jan gave so much of herself to those she supported and felt a deep responsibility to make things right in their world, or at the least, make their day a bit brighter. Over time I began to see Jan wither; her passion never waned but her faith in the system had taken its toll. She would share with me her desire to do more and be more for her clients. She would tell of the frustration she would experience as the funding wasn't there or the scope of the program she offered would change.

To her, the needs were simple, but the goal posts kept changing. Jan would promise her clients one thing one day to then have to take it away from them the next. This began to get Jan down and she contemplated leaving the sector altogether. She continued to carry the burden of feeling she was letting her clients down at a time when they needed her most.

Jan's story isn't uncommon but it's one that echoes throughout the aged care industry every day. Staff give so much and take the little that's left over for themselves. A study conducted by the Australian Nursing and Midwifery Federation released a survey of almost 1000 workers in aged care with 37% of respondents indicating they were planning to quit the sector within the next one to five years, and another 21% planning to leave within the next 12 months.

Respondents cited reasons such as 'feelings of hopelessness and abandonment' as influencing their decision. Many staff indicated they felt 'exhausted, demoralised, and resigned' (Australian Nursing & Midwifery Federation, 2022).

In an industry where staff are leaving due to burnout, it's hoped that through the creation of the Dementia Doula role, staff like Jan will not only have increased job opportunities but also feel more supported in their practice. Through the promotion of better self-awareness and self-care practices, we aim to ensure Dementia Doulas are better positioned and empowered to make the necessary changes to their personal and working lives sooner rather than later.

Supporting Dementia Doulas

At Dementia Doulas International, our team is here to support Dementia Doulas to become the Dementia Doula they were meant to be, helping them to grow into their role and making sure it's a perfect fit. We give Dementia Doulas the space and flexibility to define their own role and mission, to evolve in a way that allows their strengths and passions to emerge and become their flagship.

We provide an ongoing Dementia Doula community that provides support and encourages continued professional and personal development, inspiring new ways of thinking. It's a community that provides a forum for staying connected with other Dementia Doulas. It's also an opportunity to share in learnings, things that worked, or didn't work, along with insights and stories from the field. It's a place for celebrating the wins and sharing in the losses.

By coming together in this way, Dementia Doulas develop confidence to take steps into often unchartered territories but still know they're not alone. They can glance over their shoulder in times of uncertainty and know their Dementia Doula community will be standing there ready to offer assistance or advice when needed.

Bringing it all to life

At Dementia Doulas International, we provide education for our Dementia Doulas that's more than just improving skills and knowledge. We build on this foundation with training that's more tangible, inspirational, and experiential. We enhance a Dementia Doula's purpose and show them what's possible and what they can ultimately achieve within realistic prospects. Training for a Dementia Doula creates a baseline for practice and continues with ongoing professional and personal development essential for building recognition within the aged care sector, credibility, and self-confidence. Dementia Doulas are then best placed when working alongside health professionals to have conversations others may either be too busy or not sure how to have.

A path to new beginnings

This book, *The Dementia Doula,* has introduced and brought to life the world of the Dementia Doula. It's shone a spotlight on what the role is, where it fits and what's possible moving forward. It's brought together the components essential for role development and for enhancing the quality-of-service provision within the dementia care field. It's highlighted the importance of a specific focus on preparing for end-of-life in the dementia context. This is a book that will challenge mindsets and encourage a different way of thinking, a better way forward toward what is possible if we're prepared to look and think outside the box.

The intention is not only to provide current or prospective Dementia Doulas with a valuable resource, but also to validate the practices of those who are Dementia Doulas at heart. It will guide Dementia Doulas in their practice to provide dementia care from a place of passion and inspire others to do the same.

Through the sharing of stories, we can all support each other to be better at dementia care than we were yesterday and prepare us for being even better again tomorrow.

The Dementia Doula role is one that will inspire changes to end-of-life practices and provide opportunities for those seeking a fulfilling path. They will better prepare families to play a more connected role in care provision and remove the fear of the unknown. A Dementia Doula will ultimately lighten the load of expectation which is a weight carried unnecessarily by families. And by creating communities of collaboration and connection, the weight can be more evenly dispersed with others willing to step up and play their part.

The Dementia Doula explores the 'why'. Why the need for a Dementia Doula? Why might I be drawn to the Dementia Doula role? Why might I feel so restricted or directionless in my current practice? Why do I feel a need to do more? This book sets the scene for tackling what at face value has, in the past, seemed impossible. It provides hope through redefining Compassionate care to someone living with dementia and what that should and could look like. So, where this book is the 'why' for those who choose to take that next step, Dementia Doula training becomes the 'how'. There cannot be one without the other, otherwise we risk defaulting back into a task-focused model of care giving.

Are you the Dementia Doula difference?

Dementia Doulas provide an opportunity to challenge current thinking around dementia care and to continue building on the vision so those standing on the outside looking into our Dementia Doula community do so knowing they want and need to be a part of it. We better serve those who need it most, not by working more efficiently as individuals, but by coming together to share insights and learnings. Making dementia care a community responsibility, seeing possibilities to explore Compassionate care mixed with sprinklings of collaborative care is the next step. It's a community focus on a whole different level, going back to the village model where everyone takes responsibility for their own.

My hope is for those I've met along the way who have said, 'I'd love to do something like this but don't think I can'. May this book inspire you enough to know that you're exactly the type of person the world of dementia needs. Be encouraged to know that we are but one cog in a very big wheel and that it's essential we join with others, never losing sight of the value the Dementia Doula brings alongside other services and roles. We no longer need to feel as if something is missing, or that there's a gap in services that seems to leave people hanging, waiting for 'someone' to step forward with a reassuring hand to offer some direction.

The Dementia Doula role is not about being a separate entity operating independently. It's about filling a gap within existing services and complementing the work of others. Dementia Doulas are better placed to shoulder an emotional burden many others find too heavy to carry. I look forward to the day when we no longer ask, '*Is* there a Dementia Doula on staff?' but instead ask, 'Why *isn't* there a Dementia Doula on staff?' As Dementia Doulas we may not be able to be everything to everybody but if we stick to our vision, then together, we'll make a huge difference regardless. A better day is here for those living with a diagnosis of dementia to feel comfortable and reassured, knowing we'll be there for them when they need us most, and while we can't take dementia away, we can ensure we make someone's wishes a reality. We can make moments matter.

Jill's story ...

A colleague and I once walked into a care home we'd not visited before, and as we passed the kitchen a woman appeared through the doorway stirring a bowl of food. She spoke with a friendly voice and had a gentle smile. She politely asked who we were. We explained we'd been sent to observe the uniqueness of this specific care home model and see what made it work. She introduced herself as Jill, and she welcomed us with a sweeping gesture of the room. Jill told us we were welcome to look around and if we had any questions, anyone would be happy to help. As I thanked Jill, I asked how long she'd been working within the organisation. She laughed and said, 'Oh, I don't work here. My husband's over there. I'm just getting his lunch.'

This conversation warmed my heart. For the first time I saw what could be done. Jill felt like a genuine part of the care environment. She'd been empowered. She felt confident in initiating the care her husband needed. What Jill also had was ownership. She'd been made to feel this was her and her husband's home environment and she looked comfortable in it. Not only had she come from the kitchen, normally out of bounds to all but staff, but she questioned two intruders walking in unannounced and politely asked our reason for being there.

Jill's story is a sign of things slowly starting to happen, change happening for the better, the long-awaited shift in thinking. What this means for us as Dementia Doulas is the need to keep the momentum going and remembering all that's now possible.

Question for reflection ...

Are you a voice for those without? Could you be the Dementia Doula difference?

The gift ...

By uniting as one, we have the power to create a shift there'll be no turning back from.

When working with a family I start by asking myself what the family needs from me rather than what I can do for them.

• Dementia Doula •

Notes on Sources

1. Where there's a written will there's a way

Swerissen, H & Duckett, S (2014), 'Dying Well': pp.1-37
https://grattan.edu.au/report/dying-well/

Crowther, J., Wilson, K., Horton, S. & Lloyd-Williams, M. (2013), 'Palliative care for dementia—time to think again?': Q J Med, vol 106, pp.491–494

2. Filling the empty seat at the table

Fox, S., FitzGerald, C., Harrison Dening, K, Irving, K, Kernohan, W.G., Treloar, A., Oliver, D., Guerin, S. and Timmons, S. (2018), 'Better palliative care for people with a dementia: summary of interdisciplinary workshop highlighting current gaps and recommendations for future research': BMC Palliative Care, vol 17:9, pp.1-11

Dementia Australia – Help Sheet (2022),
https://www.dementia.org.au/sites/default/files/helpsheets/Helpsheet-AboutDementia01-WhatIsDementia_english.pdf

Dementia Australia (2022), https://www.dementia.org.au/about-dementia/dementia-research/causes-of-dementia

Dictionary.com, (2022), https://www.dictionary.com/browse/doula

Krawczyk, M. & Rush, M. (2020), 'Describing the end-of-life doula role and practices of care: perspectives from four countries': Palliative Care & Social Practice, vol. 14, pp.1–15

Rawlings, D., Tieman, J., Miller-Lewis, L., & Swetenham, K. (2018), 'What role do Death Doulas play in end-of-life care? A systematic review. In Health & Social Care in the Community': Wiley, Vol. 27: 3, pp.82– 94

3. Tailored for the perfect fit

Crowther, J., Wilson, K.C.M., Horton, S. & Lloyd-Williams, M. (2013), 'Compassion in healthcare – lessons from a qualitative study of the end of life care of people with dementia': Journal of the Royal Society of Medicine, vol. 106: 12, pp.492–497

Soklaridis S., Ravitz P., Adler Nevo G., Lieff S. (2016), 'Relationship-centred care in health: A 20-year scoping review': Patient Experience Journal, vol. 3:1, pp.130-145

Kirby Bates Associates (2018, 13 September), Fitzpatrick, M.A., '5 Essential Skills for Compassionate Care in Nursing' https://kirbybates.com/blog/5-essential-skills-for-compassionate-care-in-nursing/

Tierney, S., Seers, K., Tutton, E. & Reeve, J. (2017), 'Enabling the flow of compassionate care: a grounded theory study', BMC Health Services Research, vol 17:174, pp.1-12

4. Gaps that needed filling

Jones, K., Birchley, G., Huxtable, R., Clare, L., Walter, T. & Dixon, J., (2019), 'End-of-life Care: A Scoping Review of Experiences of Advance Care Planning for People with Dementia', Dementia, vol. 18:3, pp.825–845

van Riet Paap, J., Mariani, E., Chattat, R., Koopmans, R., Kerhervé, H., Leppert, W., Forycka, M., Radbruch, L., Jaspers, B., Vissers, K., Vernooij-Dassen, M., & Engels, Y., (2015), 'Identification of the palliative phase in people with dementia: a variety of opinions between healthcare professionals', vol. 14:56, pp.1-6

Crowther, J., Wilson, K., Horton, S. & Lloyd-Williams, M. (2013), 'Palliative care for dementia—time to think again?': Q J Med, vol 106, pp.491–494

Swerissen, H & Duckett, S (2014), 'Dying Well': pp.1-37 https://grattan.edu.au/report/dying-well/

Palliative Care Australia, 'Australian National Palliative Care Standards', 5th edition, (Canberra: PCA, 2018), PalliativeCare-National-Standards-2018_Nov-web.pdf

Palliative Care Australia, (2022), resource 'What is palliative care?', https://palliativecare.org.au/resource/what-is-palliative-care/

Victoria State Government – Department of Health, (2022), 'Palliative approach focuses on improving quality of life', https://www.health.vic.gov.au/patient-care/palliative-approach-focuses-on-improving-quality-of-life

Australian Commission on safety & quality in health care, (2022), 'End-of-life care', https://www.safetyandquality.gov.au/our-work/end-life-care

Mitchell, G., Agnelli, J., McGreevy, J., Diamond, M., Roble, H., McShane, E., Strain, J., (2016), 'Palliative and end-of-life care for people living with dementia in care homes: part 1', nursingstandard.com, vol 30:43, pp.54-60

5.   Snapshot of a better day

Mitchell, G., Agnelli, J., McGreevy, J., Diamond, M., Roble, H., McShane, E., Strain, J., (2016), 'Palliative and end-of-life care for people living with dementia in care homes: part 1', nursingstandard.com, vol 30:43, pp.54-60

6.   The weight of grief and loss

Palliative Care Australia. Joint policy statement, Palliative Care Australia and Dementia Australia (2018, May), *https://palliativecare.org.au/wp-content/uploads/dlm_uploads/2015/04/Dementia-Policy-Statement-2018_Final-New-Template.pdf*

Beyond Blue, (2022), 'Risk factors for older people', https://www.beyondblue.org.au/who-does-it-affect/older-people/risk-factors-for-older-people

Beyond Blue, (2022), 'Grief and loss – What are grief and loss?', https://www.beyondblue.org.au/the-facts/grief-and-loss

Beyond Blue, (2022), 'Grief and loss', https://www.beyondblue.org.au/docs/default-source/resources/bl0390-grief-loss-and-depression-fact-sheet_acc.pdf?sfvrsn=ff1646eb_2

Beyond Blue, (2022), 'Looking after yourself', https://www.beyondblue.org.au/the-facts/supporting-someone/looking-after-yourself

Better Health Channel, (2021), 'Grief - how to support the bereaved', https://www.betterhealth.vic.gov.au/health/servicesandsupport/grief-how-to-support-the-bereaved#bhc-content

Beyond, (2022), 'What is delayed grief?', https://beyond.life/help-centre/grief-loss-bereavement/what-is-delayed-grief/

Flinders University, (2022), 'Accidental counselling', https://ienrol.flinders.edu.au/index.php/course/ACCCN

7. Preparing for a better tomorrow

Martyr, A., Nelis, S., Quinn, C., Wu1, Y., Lamont, R., Henderson, C., Clarke, R., Hindle, J.V., Thom, J., Jones, I., Morris, R., Rusted, J., Victor, C. & Clare, L. (2018), 'Living well with dementia: a systematic review and correlational meta-analysis of factors associated with quality of life, well-being and life satisfaction in people with dementia', Psychological Medicine, vol 48, pp.2130–2139

Dementia & Sensory Challenges leaflet, Highland Print and Design. Distributed by Dementia Centre.

Plett, H. (2015), 'Art of hosting, circle, Community, Compassion, grace, grief, journey, leadership', https://heatherplett.com/2015/03/hold-space/

8. Building a collaborative community

Bivins, R., Tierney, S., & Seers, K. (2017), 'Compassionate care: not easy, not free, not only nurses', BMJ Qual Saf, vol. 26 pp.1023–1026

Edberg, Bird, Richards et. al., (2008), 'Strain in nursing care of people with dementia: Nurses' experience in Australia, Sweden, and UK', Aging and Mental Health, vol. 12, pp.236-243).

Soklaridis S., Ravitz P., Adler Nevo G., Lieff S. (2016), 'Relationship-centred care in health: A 20-year scoping review': Patient Experience Journal, vol. 3:1, pp.130-145

9. Support as the end draws near

Barbato, M.P., (2005), 'Caring for the dying patient', Internal Medicine Journal, vol. 35, pp.636–637

Mogan, C., Lloyd-Williams, M., Harrison Dening, K., & Dowrick, C., (2018), 'The facilitators and challenges of dying at home with dementia: A narrative synthesis', Palliative Medicine, vol. 32:6, pp.1042–1054

Mitchell, G., Agnelli, J., McGreevy, J., Diamond, M., Roble, H., McShane, E., Strain, J., (2016), 'Palliative and end-of-life care for people living with dementia in care homes: part 2', nursingstandard.com, vol 30:44, pp.54-60

Palliative Care Australia, 'Australian National Palliative Care Standards', 5th edition, (Canberra: PCA, 2018), PalliativeCare-National-Standards-2018_Nov-web.pdf

Barbato, M, *Midwifing Death* (Michael Barbato 2013), p.19

Alzheimer's Society UK, (2021), 'End of life care', https://www.alzheimers.org.uk/sites/default/files/2018-10/531LP%20End%20of%20life%20care.pdf

Dementia Australia, Help sheet – Palliative care, (2017), https://www.dementia.org.au/sites/default/files/helpsheets/Helpsheet-CaringForSomeone21-PalliativeCare_english.pdf

10. A new path awaits

Lord, K., Livingston, G., Robertson, S., & Cooper, C. (2016), 'How people with dementia and their families decide about moving to a care home and support their needs: development of a decision aid, a qualitative study', BMC Geriatrics, vol 16:68, pp.1-8

Dementia Australia, (2022), 'Key facts and statistics', https://www.dementia.org.au/statistics

Cocker, F., & Joss, N., (2016), 'Compassion Fatigue among Healthcare, Emergency and Community Service Workers: A Systematic Review', International Journal of Environmental Research and Public Health, vol. 13:618, pp.1-18

Palliative Care Australia, (2022), 'Self-Care Matters', https://palliativecare.org.au/resource/resources-self-care-matters/

ANMF National Aged Care COVID-19 Survey (2022) - Final Report | March 2022, https://www.anmf.org.au/media/gigpvx4t/anmfagedcarecovid-19survey2022_finalreport.pdf

Acknowledgments

This was never just a book coming to life but also a concept, one that will continue making a difference in the lives of so many. I find myself needing to acknowledge those who have supported a vision that first started many years ago while still being a little fuzzy around the edges. The challenge was always in deciphering what this could look like and what it would ultimately become.

Firstly, to Joanne, thank you for supporting the initial concept all those years ago, things may have been very different had you not shared in the vision I was committed to bringing to life. Having someone believe in you is the greatest gift anyone can receive, and your support means more to me than you'll ever know.

To Stephen, not sure where to start, but you certainly belong on this page. Our paths crossed professionally for such a short moment in time, but meeting you put my life on a trajectory I could never have imagined. I thank you for seeing in me what I could not or refused to see in myself. I thank you for your unrelenting pushing or 'encouragement' as I think you called it. Without it I wouldn't be on the path I now find myself.

To Nina and Lorrie, what would I do without your belief and support? You are both amazing women with gifts that I so appreciate and find myself drawing on regularly. Please know I don't ever for a second take you for granted and value all you bring. Having you as part of the team, sharing in the vision means I never feel alone.

To Marie, I continue to be in awe of all you do and achieve in the world of dementia. Your gifts and dedication do not go unnoticed, and you truly make a difference in ways you will never fully comprehend. I am forever grateful having you by my side.

To my wonderful husband John and amazing son Louis, I am blessed to have you join me for the ride I find myself on. I couldn't do any of this without the support of you both and I know you'll never fully understand the true role you play in helping others you will unlikely ever have the opportunity to meet.

And lastly, I am again indebted to those who have shared and continue to trust me with their experiences. What I have discovered and been in total awe of is the families, staff and those living with dementia that willingly want to be a part of this journey, to share their stories and ensure those that follow have a smoother path than they themselves experienced. What a gift to us all to learn from those who will ultimately become our greatest teachers. They will continue to inspire us and show us the way forward. I thank you from the bottom of my heart.